DATE			

The Story of Your Foot

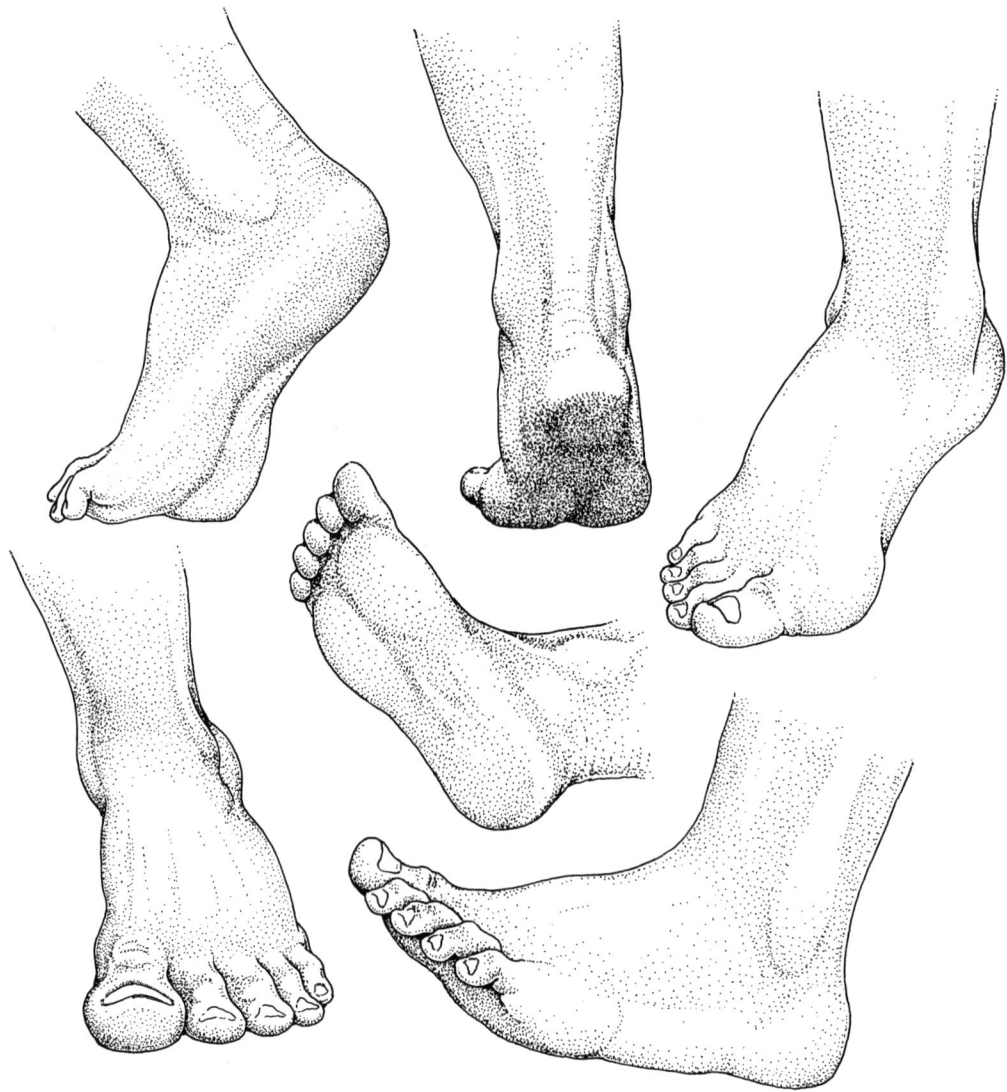

The Story of Your Foot

Dr. Alvin Silverstein and Virginia B. Silverstein

illustrated by Greg Wenzel

G. P. Putnam's Sons   New York

For Coach Robert O'Rourke

Text copyright © 1987 by Alvin and Virginia B. Silverstein
Illustrations copyright © 1987 by Greg Wenzel
All rights reserved. This book, or parts thereof,
may not be reproduced in any form without permission
in writing from the publishers. Published simultaneously
in Canada by General Publishing Co. Limited, Toronto.

Designed by Alice Lee Groton

First impression
Printed in the United States of America

Library of Congress Cataloging-in-Publication Data
Silverstein, Alvin.   The story of your foot.
Bibliography: p.   Includes index.   1. Foot—Juvenile
literature.   I. Silverstein, Virginia B.   II. Wenzel,
Gregory C.   III. Title.   QM549.S55   1987   611′.98
86-12293   ISBN 0-399-61216-5 (lib. bdg.)

Contents

1. Our Humble Servants *7*

2. Feet: The Outside Story *13*

3. Feet: The Inside Story *28*

4. Feet in Action *48*

5. Foot Fitness *62*

Index *76*

∘1∘

Our Humble Servants

If you're like the average American, you'll take a total of about 15,000 steps today, covering some four and a half miles. In a typical lifetime that comes to about 115,000 miles. And if you're a jogger or take part in some other active sport, those totals may be far higher. To move your body around over all that distance, you need a firm, flexible, and durable foundation. That foundation is provided by your two feet. With each step, those two small structures must support the entire weight of your body.

You'd think people would put a special value on two such hard-working structures as the feet. Instead, they are probably the most misunderstood, mistreated, and underappreciated organs in the body. Usually we don't even think about our feet—unless they hurt.

Normal feet shouldn't hurt; when they do, it's a sign that there is something wrong with them, or that they are being mistreated. Perhaps their design isn't perfect, but ordinarily they do an excellent job of holding us up and moving us around in an amazing variety of ways. Feet provide sturdy supports when we walk or run, whether it is on soft sand or hard pavement or uneven ground covered with ruts and loose stones. Feet are launching platforms when we jump and paddles when we swim. We do show them some consideration by covering them with shoes, socks, and other forms of footwear to keep them warm, give them extra support, and protect them from injury. But sometimes we force our feet to wear coverings that are so poorly fitting or badly designed that they are more like torture instruments than protections. When we do, we usually pay a price in pain.

The human foot is the result of millions of years of changes and compromises, in a process that scientists call evolution. An amazing variety of foot designs can be found in the animal kingdom. Some animals have a lot of feet. The champions are the millipedes, or "thousand-leggers." Actually, they don't quite live up to their name: The longest millipedes have only about five hundred legs, arranged in pairs along their wormlike bodies, but that is still a very impressive total. Spiders and their relatives have a total of eight legs; insects—from ants and houseflies to all the other insect species that swarm on our planet—have six legs. Most reptiles and mammals have four legs, each equipped with a foot at the end. Birds, when they are not flying, hop about on two feet; some flightless birds such as the ostrich have strong legs and feet and can walk, run, and kick very skillfully indeed.

Only a few species of mammals are *bipeds*—two-legged animals—and most of them cheat a little. Bears can stand and walk on their two hind legs, but they are just as likely to go about on all four legs. Kangaroos use a long, thick tail as a "third leg" to help out when they stand or leap on their heavy hind legs. Gorillas and chimpanzees, the apes that are among

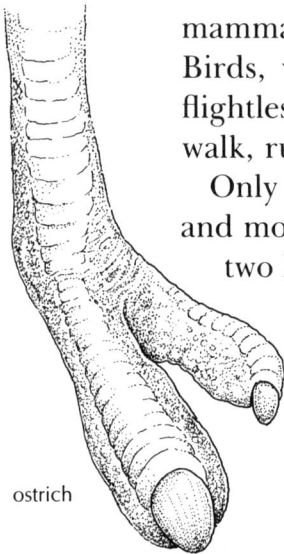

ostrich

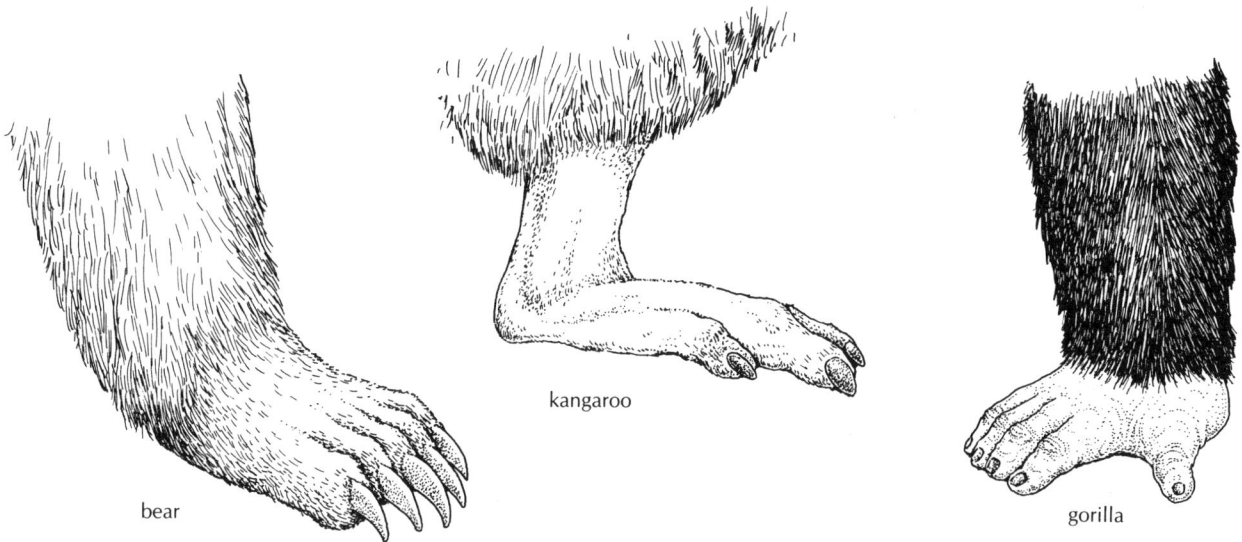

bear

kangaroo

gorilla

our closest animal relatives, walk on two legs, but they often lean on the knuckles of their hands for some extra support. Humans are the only mammals that stand, walk, and run on two feet all the time. We can do this because of the well-adapted structure of the human body, and especially the feet. Some animals, such as snails and clams, get along with only a single foot. But they cannot move as quickly or effectively as we can; they just glide along slowly.

The variety of animal feet includes a number of special multipurpose designs. Spiders sniff the air with special smelling organs on the tips of the first pair of walking legs. Butterflies taste the sweet nectar of flowers with sense organs on their forefeet. Houseflies and bees also have taste organs on their feet. Bees, in fact, are walking tool kits. The bee's front legs are

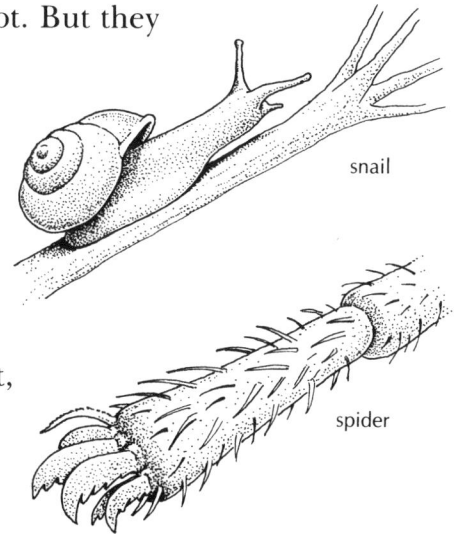

snail

spider

equipped with combs to clean her eyes and antennae. Spurs on the middle legs scrape wax from glands on the bee's abdomen. (The wax is used to build the honeycomb.) Fringes of hair on the feet of the middle and hind legs collect pollen from flowers, and on the hind legs hairs are shaped into pollen baskets to carry the pollen back to the hive.

bee

Many animals use their feet as weapons. Cats' toes are tipped by razor-sharp claws that they can keep covered in sheaths or extend like slashing knives. (Used more gently, the claws also make good fur combs in the cat's daily grooming.) Kangaroos, ostriches, and horses all can deliver deadly kicks.

Some animals use feet to pick up and hold things. Squirrels and raccoons hold food in their forefeet in much the same way that we humans use our hands. Parrots can perch with one foot and hold a piece of fruit in the other. The variety of animal feet also includes specialized shovels, paddles, snowshoes, climbing equipment, hooks, suction disks, and even "glue feet." (Have you ever wondered how a fly can walk upside down on the ceiling? Its feet have moistened hairs that stick to the surface.)

Some people can pick up marbles with their toes, or learn to dress themselves, eat, and even write and draw pictures with their feet. For most of us, though, feet perform only their one main job of holding us up while we stand and move around. They are well adapted for that job, and scientists believe that adaptation was a key part of the process of evolution that produced the first humans.

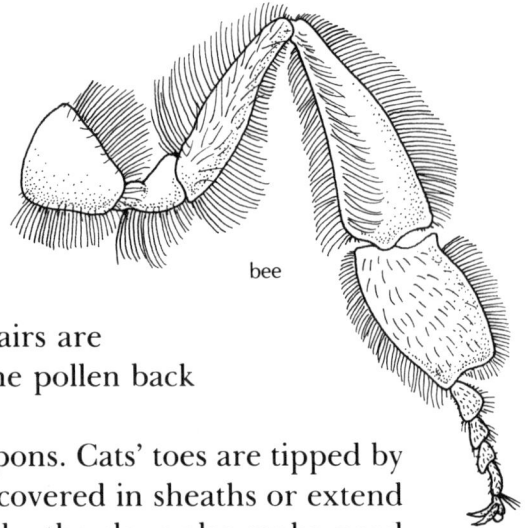

Our closest living relatives, the monkeys and apes, as well as the fossils of creatures that lived millions of years ago, provide clues to how we humans evolved. Monkeys do not really have distinct hands and feet, as we do. Instead, they have two pairs of what might be called foot-hands. These foot-hands have long, nimble fingers and thumbs that are good for picking up objects and manipulating them—just like hands. They also have long, thick, cushiony palm pads that form a kind of heel—just like feet. The monkey can use these foot-hands—any one of them—to swing from a branch or pluck a piece of fruit and hold it for eating. Down on the ground monkeys walk on all fours, with their foot-hands flat on the ground. The apes have forelimbs that are true hands, without the monkeys' footlike heels. But even apes use their hands part-time to get around, swinging from tree branches or propping themselves up on the ground with their knuckles.

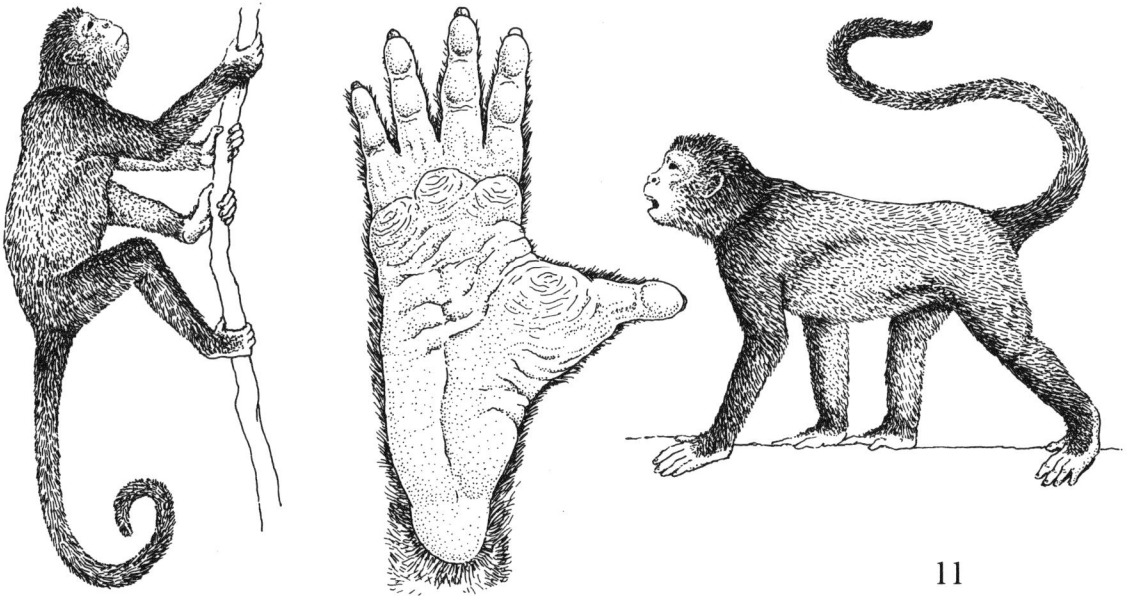

Fossil bones show that a few million years ago new kinds of apelike creatures appeared on the earth. Their brains were larger, and their bodies were built for walking upright on two legs all the time, not just for a few short steps. This change freed their hands for an almost unlimited variety of tasks. They could gather food and carry it back to their homes. They could carry their babies securely. They could make and use tools and weapons and take them along on the hunt. Among the descendants of the pre-humans, the ones with the largest brains and the best ideas about how to use their hands were the most likely to survive. Eventually true humans appeared. And feet were the foundation for it all.

In the chapters that follow, we'll find out more about the story of our feet—what they are, how they work, and how we use and abuse them.

∘ 2 ∘

Feet: The Outside Story

Feet seem rather small structures to be the foundation for the whole body. A six-foot-tall man will typically have feet that measure only about twelve inches in length; a child's feet are even smaller in proportion to the size of the body. Part of the reason feet work so well not only as supports but also as springboards and shock absorbers lies in their shape and structure. Another important part of the foot story is found beyond it, in the complex system of bones, muscles, and nerves that can move the foot or lock it firmly in place.

Although human feet may vary in details of size, shape, and color, they all follow the same basic plan. Forming approximately a right angle with the end of the leg, each foot is an elongated structure, somewhat flattened on the bottom, which points forward and ends in five *toes* that look like short, stubby fingers. That resemblance is not accidental: Remember that both our hands and our feet evolved from the original foot-hands of our monkeylike ancestors. If you examine your foot more closely, you will find many similarities to your hands. The toe on the inner side of the foot, for example, is much larger and broader than the other toes. With its wide, flat nail it looks a good bit like a thumb. And like the thumb, it has only two distinct parts, connected by a joint like a hinge. The other toes, smaller and slenderer, each have three separate parts, connected by hinge joints. The long middle part of the foot is similar to the main part of the hand, but the *heel* of the foot is a much thicker fleshy pad than the one on the hand. The bottom surface of the foot is called the *sole,* and the upper surface is the *instep.* If you look carefully at the sole of the foot, you will find that (at least, in most people) it is not perfectly flat, even in a standing position when the full weight of the body is pressing down on it. Instead, it arches upward so that the weight rests mainly on the heel and the front part of the foot, just before the toes. (That weight-bearing front part is called the *ball of the foot.*) The foot is connected to the leg by a joint called the *ankle.* Looking at your ankle, you can see two bulges, one on the outside of the leg and one

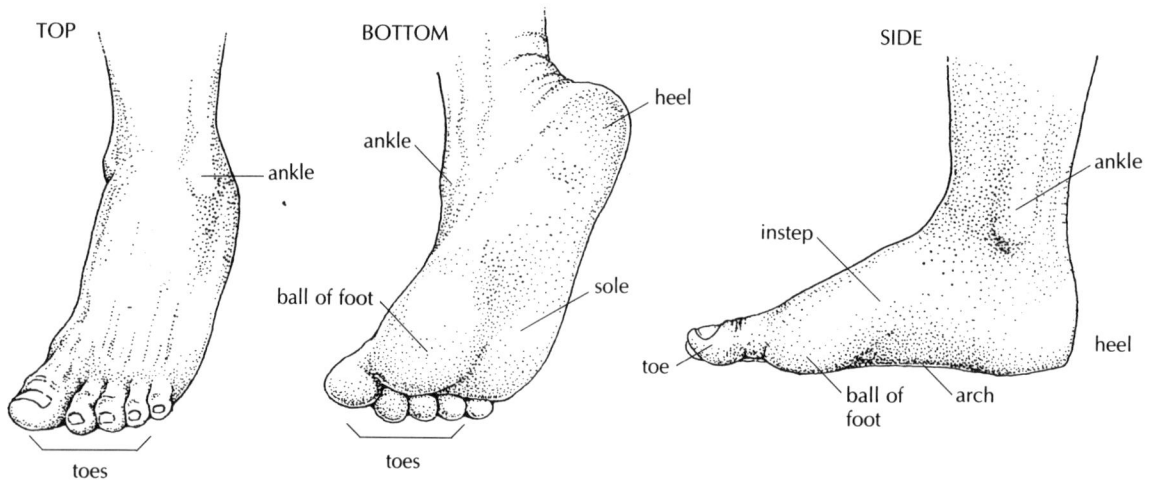

on the inside. If you feel them, they will seem very hard. The bulges are the knobby ends of the two leg bones, and the fleshy covering over them is very thin—you can get a painful bruise if you bump one of them.

Like hands, feet come in pairs. Your two feet, like your two hands, are very similar but they are not exact copies of each other. Instead, they are near mirror images, and they may have minor differences in size and shape. It is quite normal for one foot to be larger than the other. For the majority, the right foot is the larger one, but for many people it is the left. There is not necessarily any correspondence between the difference in foot size and a person's handedness. (One of us, for example, is a right-hander with a larger left foot.) People do tend to have a dominant foot, though, just as they have a dominant hand. (Which foot do you use to kick a ball?) Usually the dominant foot and hand are both on the same side of the body, but this is not always the case.

There is some disagreement about how the fingers of the hand should be named and numbered, but fortunately everybody agrees on how to count the toes of the foot. You start with the big toe on the inner side of the foot (which is usually called just that: the *big toe*) and count toward the outside of the foot. The middle toes are called by their numbers, *second, third,* and *fourth toes*. The last (and smallest) toe is called the *little toe*.

The foot is covered with a smooth and flexible coat of skin, except for the tops of the toe-tips, which are protected by flattened, horny, oval-shaped toenails. Skin is an amazing structure—a self-repairing, self-renewing covering that is made up of a number of layers. The outermost layer, the part that we see, is actually dead! It consists of dead cells, perhaps twenty deep or more, that have

SECTION OF SKIN

sebaceous gland

sense receptors

hair follicle

nerve

sweat gland

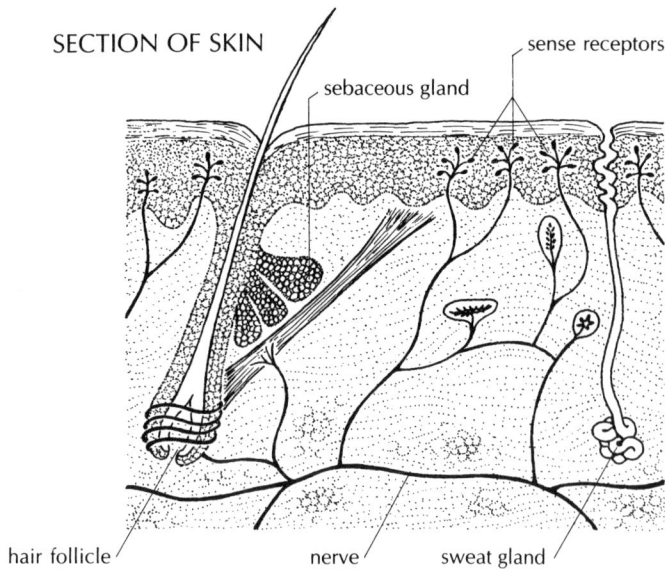

become flattened, tough, and horny. This layer of skin is called the *corneal layer,* from a word that means "horny." The horny texture comes from a protein called *keratin,* which also forms the substance of hair and nails. The dead cells of the corneal layer protect the delicate living cells from injury, from drying out, and from attacks by germs and harmful chemicals. In addition to the physical barrier it presents, the surface of the skin is slightly acid, which provides additional protection against microbes. Under this outer layer lie four layers of living cells; together with the corneal layer, they make up the *epidermis,* the outer coat of the skin.

An epidermal cell has a life of about four weeks. It starts out at the bottom of the epidermis, as a soft, slim column of living matter. (Most new skin cells are formed in the middle of the night, while you are sleeping quietly and the body's energies are not needed for other activities.) As new cells are continually formed under it, the epidermal cell moves upward through the layers, gradually flattening out until it is shaped like a flat paving stone. It produces keratin and becomes tough and horny; eventually it dies and takes its place in the corneal layer. The dead cell continues to move upward as new cells are formed underneath it and older cells flake off and are lost from the outer surface of the skin. Finally it too reaches the surface and then, in a scratch or a rub, it is gone.

Underneath the epidermis lies the true skin, the *dermis*. Its upper layer contains tiny fingerlike structures called *papillae*, which poke up into the epidermis. The papillae hold nerve endings that carry sense messages and tiny blood vessels that bring nourishing blood to the skin. The lower layer of the dermis is crisscrossed by a dense mat of fibers that give the skin strength and resilience. Most of the fibers are made of a tough, strong protein called *collagen*, but there are also elastic fibers that help to make the skin "stretchy," so that it always covers the foot and other body parts smoothly, no matter how they bend and twist.

The dermis contains a variety of structures, including sweat glands, hair follicles, oil-producing sebaceous glands, and various specialized sense receptors that gather information about the world around us.

The two outer layers of the skin, epidermis and dermis, rest on a supporting base of *subcutaneous tissue*. This tissue contains many cells that produce fat, and the fatty layer acts as a cushion and insulator. On the foot, the fat pads are especially pronounced on the bottom of the heel and on other weight-bearing parts of the sole.

The skin on the soles of the feet is rather unusual. First of all, it is ten times as thick as the skin that covers other parts of the body. It is easy to understand the reason for that. Our ancestors went about barefoot, and the soles of their feet came in direct contact with whatever they walked on. The skin covering them had to be thick and tough enough to protect the feet from injury by sharp stones and durable enough to take the rubbing wear and tear of thousands of steps a day. Even now, when we normally wear shoes to protect our feet, the soles must still provide cushioning against the shocks of our steps. The soles are caught between two hard surfaces, the bones inside the feet and the ground they stand on, and their skin covering must be very tough to stand up under that kind of pressure. When you stand, the entire weight of your body is resting on your feet; when you run or jump, forces many times your body weight come crashing down on them. In people who walk barefoot, the skin of the soles becomes thicker, tougher, and more horny. Extra thick, horny outer layers, called *calluses,* may also form over parts of the foot that are subjected to especially heavy pressure, such as the heel, which takes the shock of the body weight first at each step, and the ball of the foot, where the bones inside the foot press the sole against the ground surface as the body weight shifts forward. Protective calluses may also form on the sides or tops of the toes when shoes are too tight and rub against the feet.

The skin of the soles is so thick and tough that you might expect it to be insensitive. Actually, however, it is acutely sensitive. If someone lightly brushes a feather or a fingertip along the sole of your foot, you will probably giggle and pull your foot away. That tickles! Various kinds of *sense receptors* in the skin, from simple threadlike nerve endings to more complicated structures, gather information about touch, pressure, pain, and temperature. When they are stimulated they send a message to the brain, and you "feel." You need a continual flow of sense information from your feet to help guide you in moving about. You need to know if the surface you are walking on is soft or hard, smooth or uneven, hot or cold, so that you can adjust your stride and quicken or slow your pace if necessary. You don't normally realize how much you depend on your foot sensations until one of your feet "falls asleep." If you happen to sit or lie in a position that presses on one of the nerves coming from the feet, that nerve temporarily stops transmitting messages. What a strange sensation that produces. You can touch your foot, and even though you can see your finger pressing into the skin, you don't feel anything. If you try to stand on the foot, it is as though you were stepping on a thick, yielding layer of foam rubber. It is hard to gauge when your foot will actually touch the floor—or if it is already touching it. If you try to walk, you may stumble. A little later, as messages start to flow along the nerve again, you have a prickly, painful "pins and needles" feeling.

Doctors use the automatic reaction, or *reflex*, to tickling the sole of the foot as a way of checking on the working of the nervous system. The normal reaction changes with age. A baby reacts by extending the big toe upward and fanning the other toes outward. This is called *Babinski's reflex*. At about eighteen months, a different kind of *plantar reflex* becomes normal. ("Plantar" is a word referring to the sole of the foot.) After that age, it is normal to react to a tickle on the sole by curling the toes and bending the front part of the foot downward, as though you were a bird perching on a branch. When an older child or an adult reacts with Babinski's reflex, it is a sign of damage to the nerves that run through the spinal cord.

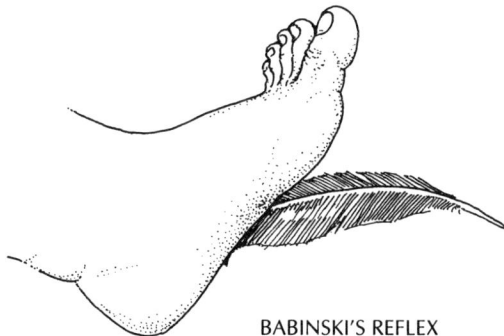

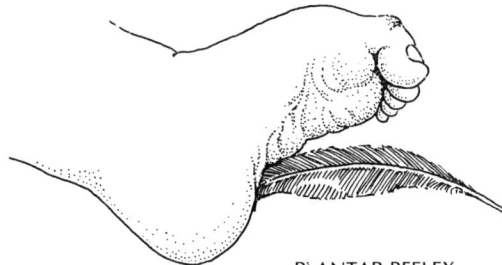

BABINSKI'S REFLEX   PLANTAR REFLEX

If you look at the sole of your foot with a magnifier, or rub ink on it and then step on a piece of paper to make a *footprint,* you will notice that the sole is covered with a pattern of swirly and crisscrossing lines. This pattern is formed by folds of epidermis lying over the ridges of papillae in the dermis. You probably know that a person's fingerprints are individual and can be used for identification. But did you know that footprints are also unique? Your own footprints form a pattern that is shared by no other human who has ever lived. Not even identical twins have the same footprints. Probably the first record of you that was ever made was a footprint. In the hospital, right after you were born, the sole of your tiny foot was pressed against an inkpad and then onto a sheet of paper, right next to your mother's fingerprint. That way, there would be no danger of your being mixed up with another baby and given to the wrong mother. (Hospitals make a print of a newborn baby's foot rather than the fingers because it is larger and the print is easier to obtain; an infant's hands are often curled in tightly.)

NORMAL   FLAT FOOT

The papillary ridges that form the footprint make a handy form of identification, but that is not their function in the body. They give the sole of the foot better gripping power. Working like the treads of a tire, they help to keep the foot from slipping when you take a step. Tiny coiled tubes in the dermis, the *sweat glands,* produce a watery secretion that adds to the sole's gripping power. This

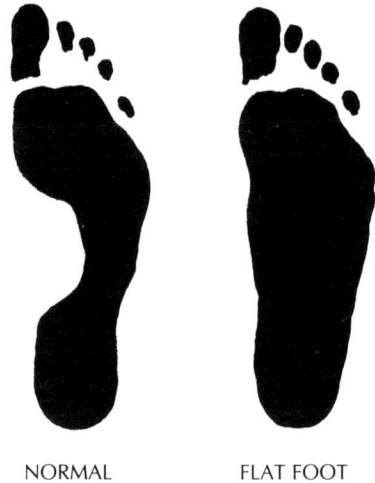

watery sweat oozes out to the surface through tiny openings called sweat pores and causes the papillary ridges to swell and grip better. If you look very closely at the skin of the sole through a magnifier, you may see some of the tiny sweat pores dotted along the papillary ridges. There are more than 200,000 sweat pores in a square inch of skin on the sole of the foot. A little sweat helps the feet to grip, but too much can make them slippery. It can also have other harmful effects. Excess sweat makes the skin on the feet soft and moist and also washes away the protective acid coating, thus creating ideal conditions for bacteria, viruses, and other microbes to grow. Germs working on the chemicals in sweat can make feet smelly, and they may invade the skin and cause painful infections. Sweat can also wash out chemicals from socks and shoes, which is bad in two ways: it eats away the insides of the shoes, and the chemicals may irritate the skin of the feet and cause rashes or sores. Various things can make the feet sweat more. One is heat—either hot weather or the heat produced by muscle action and friction during running. (Sweating is one of the body's main ways of getting rid of excess heat, which is carried away by the water.) Strong emotions can also produce sweating in certain parts of the body, including the palms of the hands and the soles of the feet. You may have noticed that your hands and feet get sweaty when you are nervous or frightened or very excited. You can minimize the bad effects of sweaty feet by wearing cotton or wool socks; their fibers draw moisture away from the surface of the foot and help it evaporate. Evaporation is aided by leather shoes that can "breathe"; synthetic materials used in some socks, stockings, and shoes trap moisture and keep feet damp and uncomfortable.

One thing that is not found on the soles but may be seen on other parts of the feet is hair. A coat of hair is rather slippery and would make walking more difficult if it covered the soles. Hair on the feet is usually rather sparse and tends to occur in patches, often on the tops of the toes. Hair is mostly made of keratin, the horny protein formed by epidermal cells. Hairs are cylinders made of three layers of keratin. The outermost layer forms tiny overlapping scales, which you can see if you look at a hair under a microscope. The color of hair is produced by a dark chemical called *melanin,* which is the same chemical that gives a dark color to skin. (Some people have naturally darker skin than others; their epidermal cells produce more melanin. Skin cells can also step up their melanin production when they are exposed to the sun, producing a suntan that helps to screen out harmful rays.) Each hair grows in a *follicle,* a sheath of living epidermal cells that tunnel down into the dermis. The bottom of the follicle is widened and rounded like the bulb of an onion and contains the root of the hair. The root is the only part of the hair that is alive. Each hair grows for a while, then stops. After a time the bulb-shaped root dies, comes loose from the follicle, and the hair falls out. Then a new hair grows out from the bottom of the follicle. Hair grows at varying rates at different ages and on different parts of the body. The hair on the head can reach a length of about five feet, but the hairs on the feet grow more slowly and are replaced after a much shorter time, so they are usually only a fraction of an inch long. A small *sebaceous gland* opens into the hair follicle. The oil that it produces helps to keep the hair and the surrounding skin smooth and supple. There are also sebaceous glands on the nonhairy parts of the foot, to help keep the skin from drying out and cracking.

Horny keratin is also the main ingredient of the *nails,* the tough, transparent plates that cover the upper surface of the toe-tips. Like hairs, a nail has a living root, which is hidden under the skin at the base of the nail. It grows out over the *nail bed,* a plate of living tissue with a rich blood supply. The pink color of toenails comes from the blood vessels showing through. If you drop something on your toe, or someone steps down hard on it, the nail bed may be damaged and may bleed. The blood clots that form make a part of the nail look black. Runners may also suffer this kind of damage to the nails when their toes jar against the fronts of too tightly fitting shoes. If you lose your whole nail in an accident, it can still grow back as long as the root is undamaged. Unlike hairs, nails grow continuously throughout a person's life. But they grow very slowly: It takes about six months to a year to replace a lost toenail.

In various cultures people have cultivated long fingernails as a mark of beauty or high rank. But growing long toenails has never been a popular fashion. When toenails are allowed to grow out uncut, if they do not break or tear off, they become extremely tough and horny and curve under as they grow. Surgeon Richard Seltzer tells of meeting a ragged old derelict in the public library. The man was hobbling about as though each step caused him great pain. Seltzer volunteered to take a look at his feet in the rest room, thinking that as a doctor he might be able to do something to help. The problem turned out to have a simple solution: The old man's toenails had grown so long and tough that they had curled under and were cutting into the soles of his feet. No great surgical skill

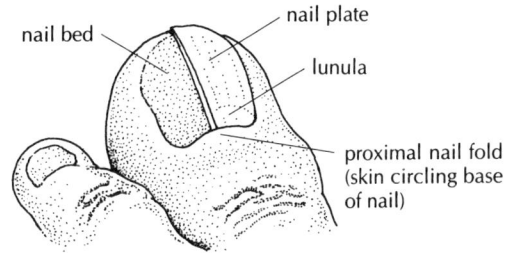

was needed to correct the problem; a pair of heavy-duty nail clippers did the job. In general, foot doctors recommend that toenails should be kept neatly trimmed, cutting them straight across, a little longer than the tips of the toes.

Toenails can act as mirrors of the body's health. Some serious circulatory and respiratory diseases may make the nails brittle or produce other telltale changes. Diabetes, psoriasis, and certain other diseases may produce ridges across the nail. These ridges are the result of abnormal growth of the *matrix*, the portion of the nail plate that grows out from the root. Tuberculosis and lung cancer can cause a general thickening of the nails. But if only one or two nails are thickened, that is usually the result of an injury or a fungus infection.

Although the feet of a newborn baby are fully formed, complete with toes and toenails, they are still very tiny and weak and not really ready to work yet. The bones and muscles that form their inner framework and moving mechanisms continue to grow and develop after birth and gradually produce some changes in the appearance of the foot, too. An infant's feet tend to point straight downward from the ends of the legs, without forming an angle at the ankle joint. (If you've ever tried to put a pair of shoes on a baby brother or sister, you can appreciate this. "Push," you urge, but the baby doesn't seem to have any real idea of how to make its heel stick out and fit into the back of the shoe.) Gradually, as the growing baby begins to pull itself up and stand, then take the first tottering steps, it learns to bend the foot up at the ankle to make a stable platform. (A child begins to walk when its body and brain reach the right stage of development, usually some time between twelve and eighteen months. Babies shouldn't be rushed into walking; they are

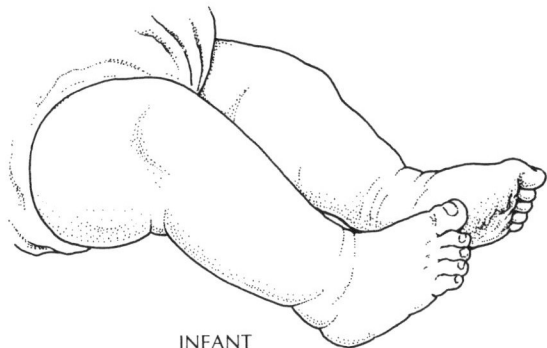

INFANT

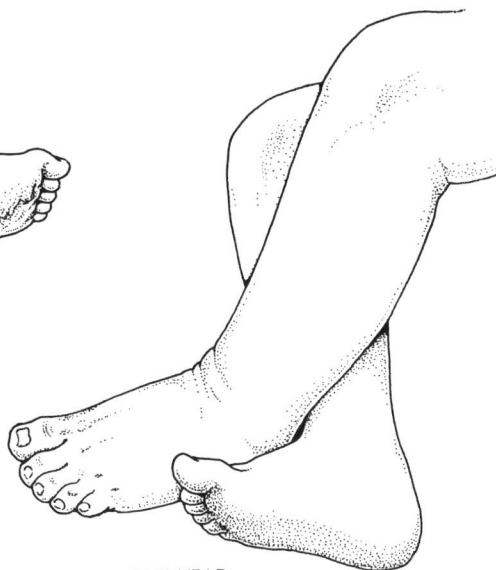

ONE YEAR

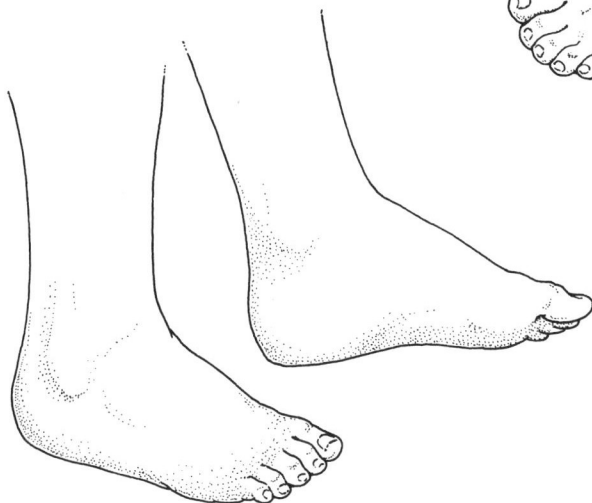

FIVE YEARS

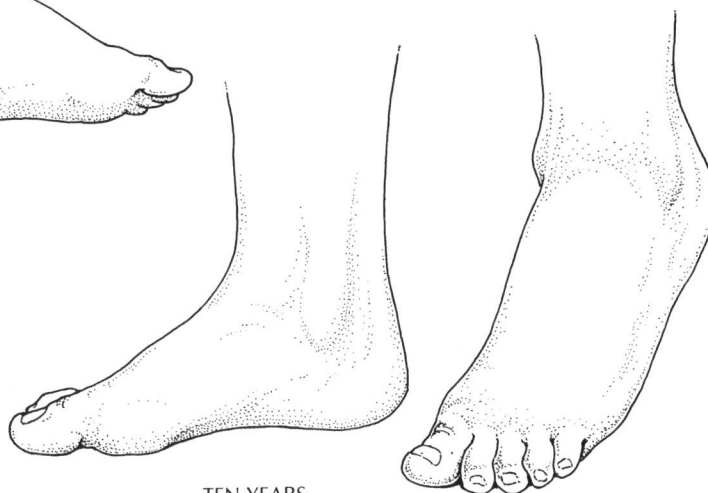

TEN YEARS

25

following their own inner timetables.) The young child's feet look flat at first, because of thick fat pads in the sole. But this "baby fat" is lost by about the age of three, and then a distinct arch can be seen unless there is some inner structural problem. The feet continue to slim down and lengthen out until they reach their full growth, some time in the teen years.

Sometimes—about once in each thousand births—the foot does not develop properly, and it is twisted out of shape or position. This condition, called *clubfoot*, can cause difficulties in walking if it is not treated. Fortunately, most clubfoot problems can be corrected very well with a combination of casts, splints, and braces, if the treatment is begun soon after birth. If not, the foot can be repaired by surgery later in life.

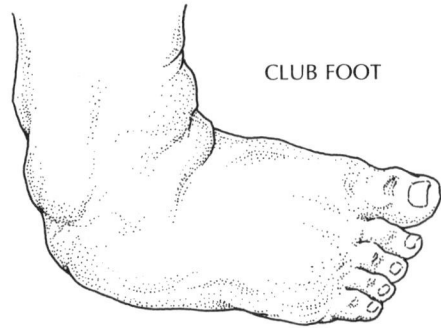

CLUB FOOT

It seems strange and sad that some cultures have produced foot defects deliberately, crippling people in a misguided quest for beauty. For more than a thousand years, Chinese mothers tightly bound their daughters' feet, starting at about the age of five. The goal was to produce the "lotus foot," a tiny stunted structure with the front part of the foot and the heel forced close together, a high instep, and a deep cleft in the sole. By the time a woman with bound feet was an adult, the distorted structure of her feet had hardened into place. She was unable to walk normally, but hobbled along painfully, swaying in what was called the "willow walk." Why were so many generations of women willing to put up with so much disability and pain? The fashion was popular mainly because the

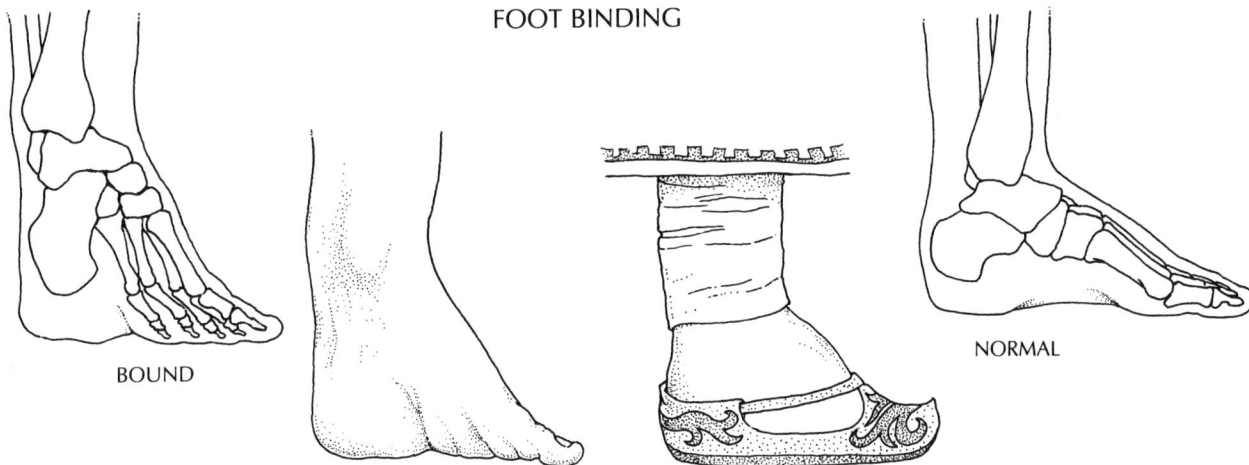

FOOT BINDING

BOUND

NORMAL

Chinese men found the willow walk very attractive. It was also a status symbol, showing that the woman's family was so wealthy that she didn't have to do any sort of physical labor but would always have people to take care of her. (Peasant women who had to work in the fields did not have bound feet.)

Foot binding was not stopped until this century, and today we find the practice barbaric. And yet in our own culture, women are willing to squeeze their feet into shoes that are too small, or wrongly shaped, with heels so high that the wearers totter along in their own version of the willow walk—just so that they can look stylish and sexy. Sometimes they pay a heavy price for their fashion, in foot problems. Attitudes may be changing, though. In 1985, actress Cybill Shepherd struck a blow for "Foot Liberation" when she attended the Emmy awards ceremony wearing a fashionable strapless evening gown with a pair of comfortable running shoes.

·3·

Feet: The Inside Story

When you think of a foundation, you normally think of something firm and solid. Feet have to provide a firm and solid foundation for your body when you stand; but they also have to act as dynamic machines, capable of complicated movements, continually pushing off against the weight of the body and molding themselves to new surfaces when you walk or run. A firm and solid inner structure would be useful for feet that spent all their time just standing around, but it would not have the flexibility needed for rapid and graceful movements. The inner structure of the human foot is made up of twenty-six separate *bones,* lashed together by tough, cordlike *ligaments.* When movement is needed, the bones can be worked like levers by the force of muscles that link them to one another and to the long bones of the leg. When solid support is needed, muscles can lock the bones of the foot together firmly, working in cooperation with the systems of muscles, bones, and nerves that hold the body upright in a complicated balancing act.

The twenty-six bones of the foot can be divided into three groups. First there are the seven foot bones or *tarsal bones,* which form the solid inner foundation of the back part of the foot. They are shaped like irregular stones, fitted together like pieces of a puzzle. The highest one is the *talus*, or ankle bone. It fits against the ends of the long bones of the lower leg (the tibia and fibula) in a joint like a hinge. This ankle joint permits you to move your whole foot up and down, bending it up at the ankle and stretching it out to point your toe. Fitted under the talus is the *calcaneus*, the heel bone. This is a large, heavy bone, and it is very strong. It has to be—when you take a step, the full weight of your body comes down on the heel. The next tarsal bone, just in front of the talus, is the *navicular* (boat-shaped), and below it is the *cuboid* (cube-shaped). Moving forward along the foot we come to the last of the tarsal bones, the three *cuneiforms* (wedge-shaped).

The next group of bones in the feet is made up of the five *metatarsals*. "Meta-" means beyond or between; the metatarsus is the middle part of the foot, between the tarsus and the toes. The metatarsals are all miniatures of the long bones, each with a narrow shaft and knobby ends. The back ends of the metatarsals are connected to the front four bones of the tarsus: the cuboid and cuneiform bones.

Each metatarsal is connected at its front end to a set of toe bones or *phalanges*. (A single toe bone is called a *phalanx*.) All together, there are fourteen phalanges in each foot. Each toe has a total of three phalanges, except for the big toe, which has only two. And the phalanges of the big toe are broader and heavier than those of the other toes. The phalanges correspond to the sections of the toes that can be seen from outside.

The bones of the foot are not firmly glued together. Instead, they are connected by joints that permit the bones to move. The movements that occur between tarsal bones are gliding move-

THE BONES OF THE FOOT

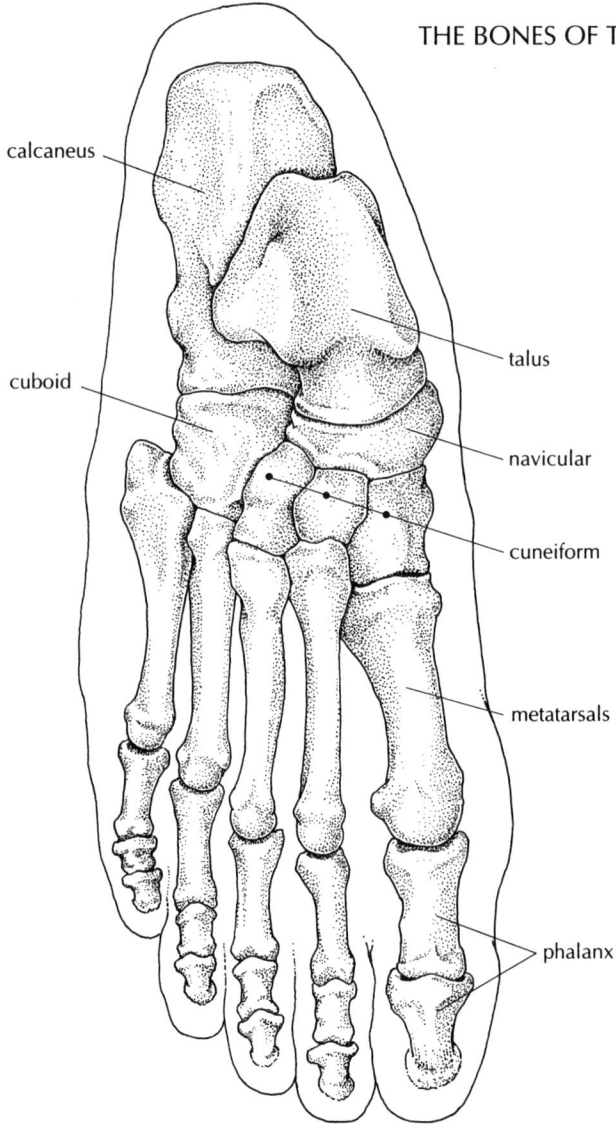

calcaneus

talus

cuboid

navicular

cuneiform

metatarsals

HAND BONES
FOR COMPARISON

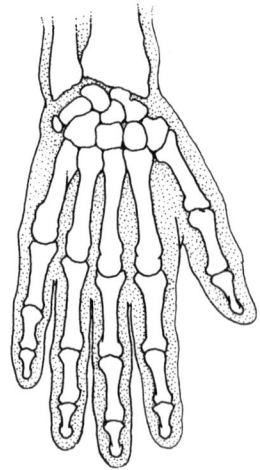

phalanx

30

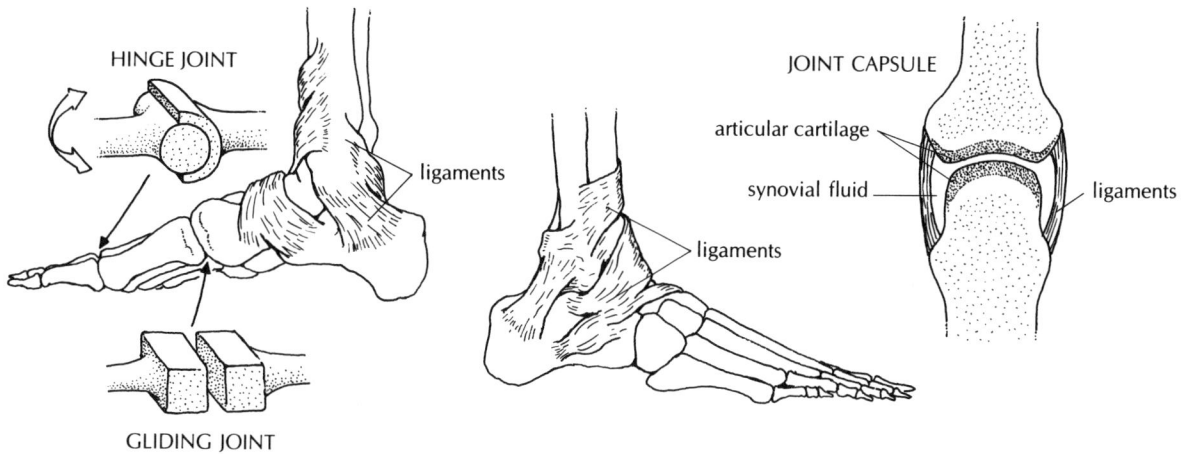

HINGE JOINT

GLIDING JOINT

ligaments

ligaments

JOINT CAPSULE

articular cartilage

synovial fluid

ligaments

ments. The phalanges are connected by hinge joints that permit back-and-forth movement. On the outside of the toes you can see knuckles, which are the hinge joints between phalanges. The hinge joints between the metatarsals and phalanges permit not only back-and-forth but also a little sideways movement, when you spread your toes. The ends of the bones are covered with soft, gristly *cartilage,* which keeps them from grinding together when the feet move. The whole joint is enclosed in a tough case called a *capsule.* Inside it the space around the bones is filled with a watery fluid that acts as a shock-absorbing cushion.

When you look at an X ray of the human foot, it looks a little strange. The toes seem to be too long. Actually, the bones that look like "toes" on the X ray are not just the phalanges but the connecting long bones of the metatarsals as well. In a living foot, you don't see the separate metatarsals because they are solidly covered by layers of muscle and skin, forming the middle of the foot.

An X ray of the hand looks very much like the one of the foot,

31

with the same kind of arrangement of pebblelike bones fitted together into a sort of mosaic and five long digits fanning out from them. There are just a few main differences. The group of wrist bones (carpals) comes to a total of eight, one more than the ankle bones (tarsals). The carpals are smaller than the tarsals, and they do not include a big heavy bone that corresponds to the heel bone. And finally, instead of all the fingers lining up the way the toes do, the thumb goes off at an angle and is connected to the carpals through a special kind of saddle joint that permits it not only to move back and forth and sideways but also to rotate. In other words, it can swing around and meet the fingers in a gripping motion. You can't grip things that way with your big toe, although you can pick up objects by clamping them between your big toe and second toe in a sort of scissors grip. You can also curl your toes around things.

There is another important difference in the arrangement of the foot bones and that of the hand bones. The bones of the feet form three distinct arches. One, the *medial arch,* runs down the inner side of the foot, from the calcaneus to the end of the first metatarsal. This is the longest and highest arch of the foot. The *lateral arch,* which runs from the calcaneus to the fifth metatarsal on the outside of the foot, is not as long or as high as the medial arch. The third arch, the *transverse arch,* runs across the foot, under the metatarsals. As you take a step and transfer the body weight to the ball of the foot, the transverse arch flattens out a little and the front of the foot spreads out, gaining more than a centimeter in width.

As you take a step, the weight of the body is transmitted first from the long bones of the leg down the ankle bone (talus) to the

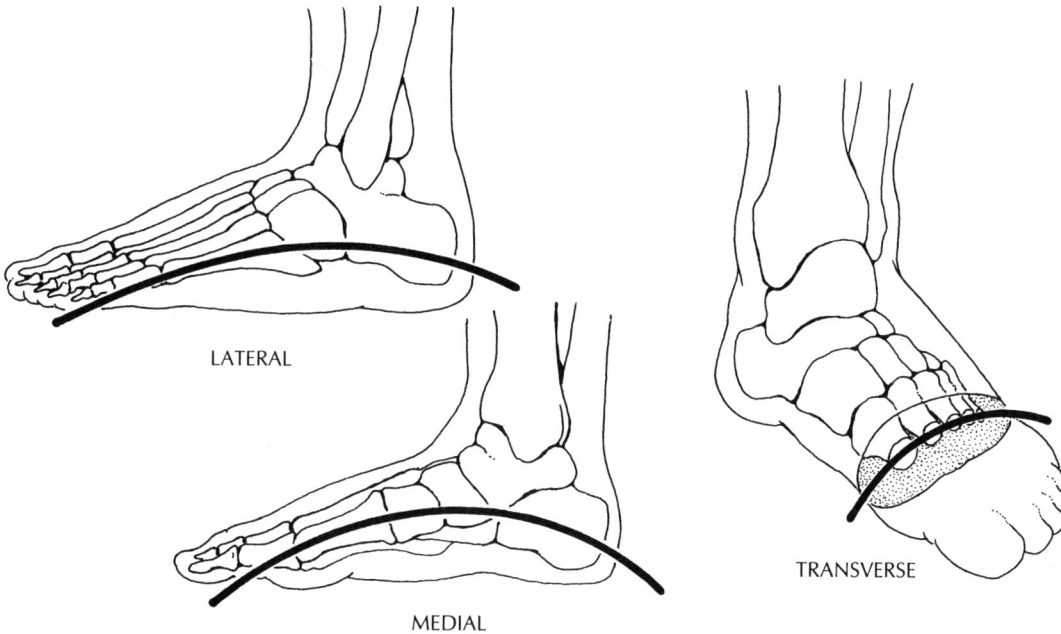

LATERAL

MEDIAL

TRANSVERSE

heel bone (calcaneus). Then, as you push off for the next step, the weight is transmitted through the other tarsal bones to the metatarsals, concentrating at the ball of the foot. During this sequence of movements, the outside of the foot (the calcaneus, the cuboid, and the fourth and fifth metatarsals and phalanges) stays fairly rigid and provides support, while the inside of the foot (the bones of the medial arch) absorbs shock.

Bones cannot move by themselves. All the movements of the feet, in walking, running, jumping, dancing, kicking, and swimming, would not be possible without the action of *muscles*. Muscles are made up of cells that are naturally very "stretchy." When they relax they get longer, and when they contract they get shorter. The ends of the muscles are anchored to bones by tough, whitish, non-stretchy structures called *tendons*. Tendons may look like thin ropes or broad, flat sheets; either way, they are very strong. Muscles cannot push; they can only pull. But by pulling on different parts of bones they may make a joint open or close, or they may make bones move up, down, around, or from side to side.

Often muscles work in pairs—there is one to open a joint and another to close it, or one muscle to move bones apart and another to draw them together. The muscles of the foot are no exception. There are *flexor* muscles, for example, that cause the toes to bend under, and *extensor* muscles that cause the same toes to stretch out straight. The flexors of the toes generally run along the sole of the foot and up the back of the leg, while the extensors of the toes run along the instep and up the front of the leg.

Twenty-eight separate muscles control the movements of the foot and ankle joint. A dozen of them extend up the lower leg, from the ankle to the knee. The largest muscle controlling movements of the foot is the *gastrocnemius* or *calf muscle,* running from the heel bone (calcaneus) up past the knee. The gastrocnemius is one of the strongest muscles in the body, able to withstand forces of up to one ton. It needs to be that strong: Though even the heaviest people weigh only a fraction of a ton, when you run or jump and come pounding down on your heel bones, the calf muscle must absorb forces many times the weight of your body. The gastroc-

MUSCLES OF THE FOOT

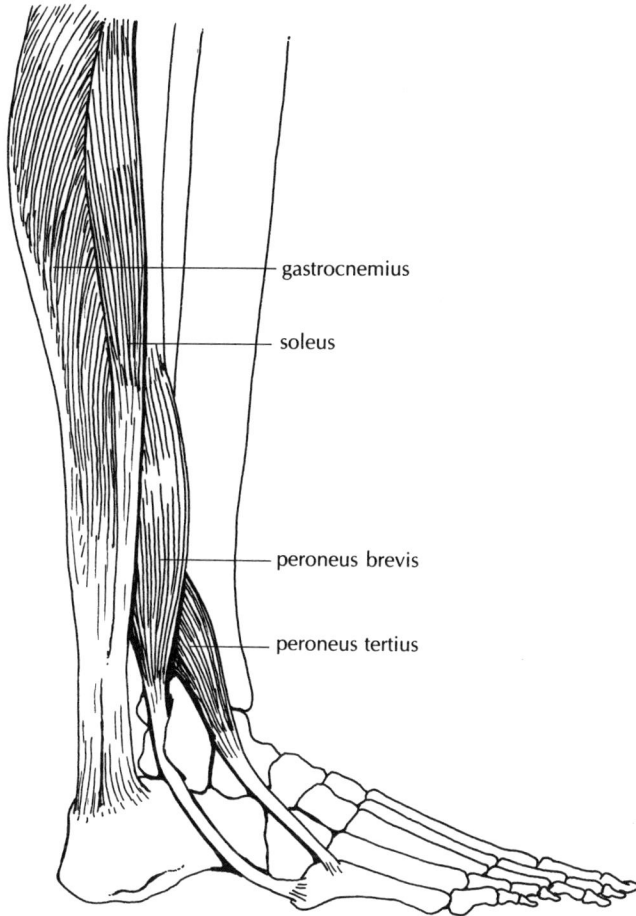

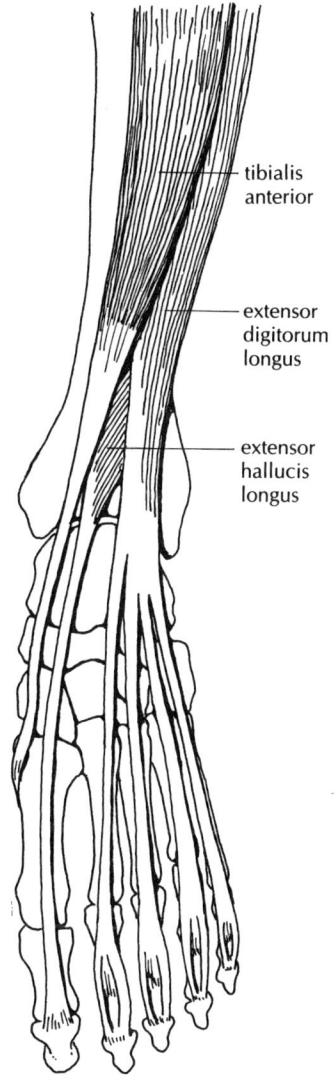

gastrocnemius

soleus

peroneus brevis

peroneus tertius

tibialis
anterior

extensor
digitorum
longus

extensor
hallucis
longus

nemius is attached to the heel bone by a thick, tough tendon called the *Achilles tendon*. If you point your toe and then bend your foot up, meanwhile feeling the back of your ankle right above the heel, you can feel this tough, cordlike tendon. (The Achilles tendon is named for an ancient Greek hero. According to the myth, when Achilles was a baby his mother dipped him into the River Styx, and its waters made him invulnerable. He grew up to become a great warrior, who could fight through the fiercest battle unharmed. But his mother had held him by the back of one heel when she dangled him in the water, and that one place, covered by her hand, did not soak up the magic powers. Eventually Achilles was killed at the battle of Troy by a wound in the back of his heel.)

The gastrocnemius makes up most of the bulging muscle you can feel at the back of the calf. Hidden underneath it is the *soleus*, another muscle attached to the heel bone by way of the Achilles tendon. The gastrocnemius contracts strongly when a person runs, while the soleus works hard during walking. Both muscles pull up on the calcaneus to bend the foot downward at the ankle joint. Other muscles in the lower leg bend the foot upward, turn it in or out, help to support the arch of the foot, and extend or bend the toes. All of them are attached to the ankle or foot bones by tendons, and so are the sixteen muscles in the foot itself. You can see some of the cordlike tendons that run from the toes across the instep to the ankle joint when you bend your toes upward as hard as you can.

If you try wiggling your toes one by one, you will discover a curious thing about the muscles that move the toes. You should be able to move your big toe with ease—up, down, and from side to side. With a bit of practice, you can also move your little toe out to the side and back again. But no matter how hard you practice, you

MUSCLES OF THE BOTTOM OF THE FOOT

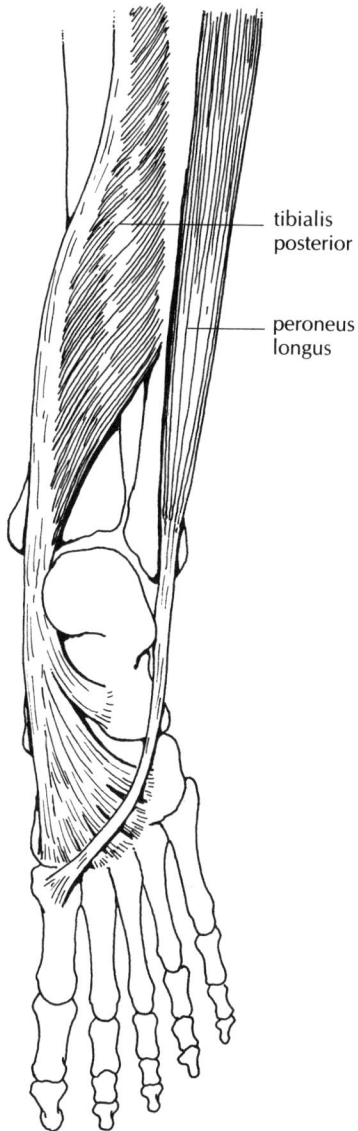

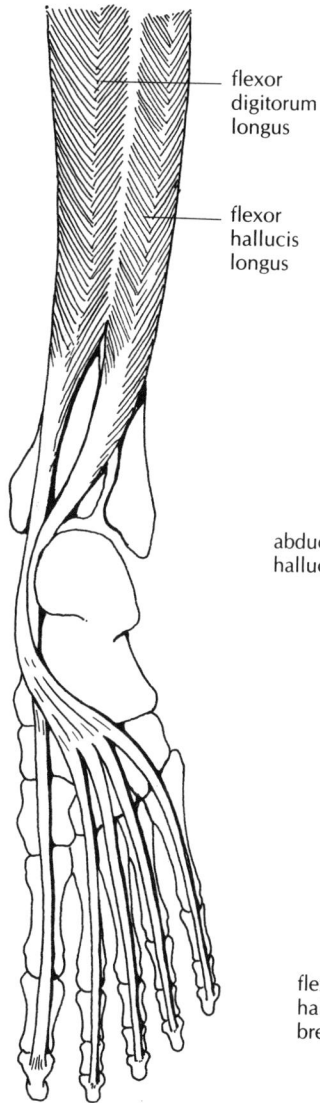

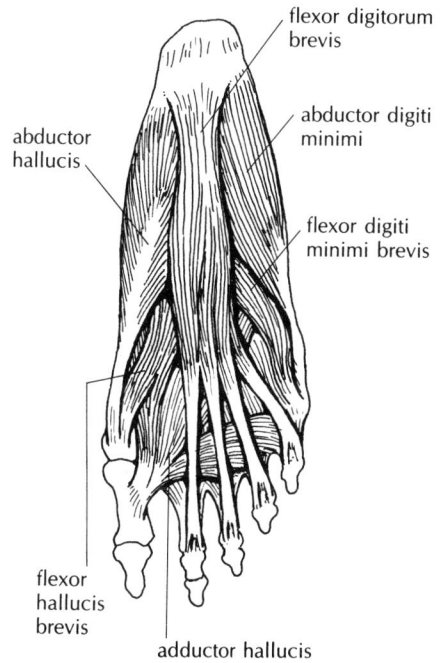

tibialis
posterior

peroneus
longus

flexor
digitorum
longus

flexor
hallucis
longus

flexor digitorum
brevis

abductor digiti
minimi

flexor digiti
minimi brevis

abductor
hallucis

flexor
hallucis
brevis

adductor hallucis

37

will not be able to move one of the middle three toes without moving the others. There is a reason for this. The big toe is provided with four separate muscles of its own, controlling three different kinds of movements: bending, moving out, and moving in. The little toe also has some muscles of its own, one to move it out and one to bend it. But all the muscles that move the middle three toes are shared among three, four, or all five toes. So none of them can move by itself.

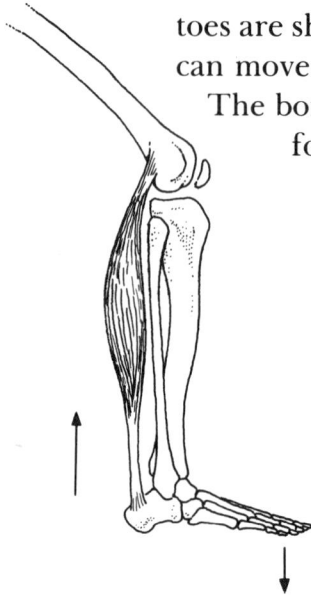

The bones of the body work like *levers,* which are moved by the forces of contracting muscles. You are familiar with some examples of levers in the world around you. A seesaw is one example: push down on one end of the board, and the other one rises. Prying open a jar lid with a spoon handle is another example of using a lever. Both in the world outside and in the body, levers are ways of changing the direction of a force or multiplying its strength.

In 1957 a Russian high jumper, Yuri Stepanov, set a new world record of seven feet one inch. Afterward, photos showed there was something unusual about the shoes the jumper was wearing. The shoe on his takeoff foot had a sole that was an inch thick and spiked in the front portion. His clever trainers were taking advantage of a law of muscle action. The special shoe lowered Stepanov's heel, which stretched his gastrocnemius muscle. But when muscles are stretched slightly, they contract with greater force. So the shoe was giving him the advantage of a stronger thrust when he started his jump. Eventually a new rule was made, outlawing the use of jumping shoes with a built-up front sole.

Muscles contract to move bones. But what makes the muscles contract? Muscles contract in response to messages carried by *nerves*. Delicate threadlike nerves connect the muscles of the feet with the spinal cord and brain.

Some nerves carry messages *to* the brain. These are *sensory nerves*. Touch, temperature, and pain receptors gather information about the world outside the body—how warm or cold it is, whether there is an object in contact with the skin, and if so, whether it is soft or hard, wet or dry, rough or smooth. They give warnings if there is something dangerous—hot enough to burn or sharp enough to cut. The foot also has some special sense receptors that gather information about what is going on inside the body. Receptors in the joints continually give the brain a picture of exactly where the various parts of the foot are and how much weight is pressing down on it. These inner cues, together with touch and pressure information from the soles of the feet, are an important part of the body's system for keeping its balance. Whenever you lift your foot or step down on it, its sense receptors provide the brain with the *feedback* it requires to plot further movements needed to keep you from falling down. There are also pain receptors to inform you when a muscle has been strained or tissues have been

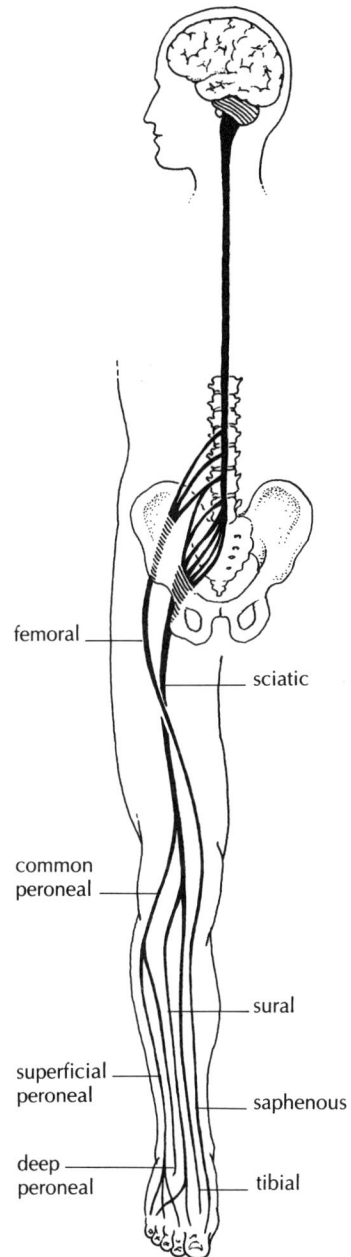

femoral

sciatic

common peroneal

sural

superficial peroneal

saphenous

deep peroneal

tibial

damaged by a cut or burn. People tend to think of pain as a bad thing, but it is actually important for the welfare of the body. If you ignore an aching muscle or a sore spot on your heel where a blister is forming, you may do more damage. Experienced athletes learn to "listen" to their bodies and ease off their activities when their feet or other body parts don't feel right.

Nerves called *motor nerves* carry messages *from* the brain and spinal cord. These are messages that tell muscles to contract and produce motion. Some actions are controlled by the spinal cord. If you dip your foot into bath water that is too hot, pain receptors in the skin signal that you are in danger of getting burned. These messages go flashing up sensory nerves to your spinal cord and from there to the brain. Before your brain has had a chance to receive and process the information—before you even realize that your foot is hurting—messages have flashed along motor nerves from the spinal cord, and you jerk your foot out of the water. A split second later, when your brain gets the message, you say "Ouch!"

Actions controlled by the spinal cord are called *reflex actions.* They are immediate, automatic responses. When someone tickles the sole of your foot, you don't consciously think about curling your toes; it happens before you have time to think. If you are expecting the tickle and concentrate very hard, you can stop yourself from reacting. But that takes a great deal of conscious effort, whereas the normal plantar reflex seems effortless.

Reflex actions, controlled by the spinal cord, are usually rather simple actions. When you are yanking your foot back out of a hot tub, you don't move it to anywhere in particular, just away, as

40

receptors in skin

interneuron   afferent neuron

effector in muscle

efferent neuron

spinal cord

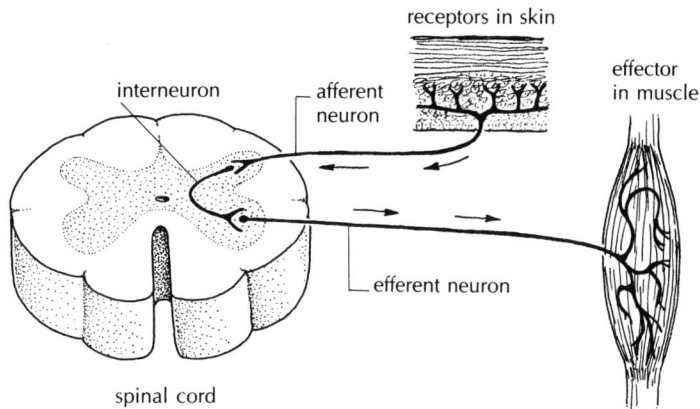

quickly as possible. But the actions controlled by the brain can be very precise and finely coordinated. Two parts of the brain are concerned with controlling the actions of muscles: the *cerebrum* (the thinking brain), which directs the actions; and the *cerebellum,* a structure at the back of the brain, which coordinates movements. When you decide to go up a flight of stairs, the cerebrum sends out signals that make muscles contract to lift your foot, swing it forward, and then put your weight on it. Signals carried along nerves from the cerebellum tell the muscles how much to contract and when to stop, so that you don't stub your toe on the front of the step, or miss the step entirely when you try to put your foot down on it.

There is something surprising about the way the nerves that carry messages to and from the brain are connected. Most of these nerves cross over to the opposite side at the bottom of the brain. So the left side of the brain receives messages about what is happening on the right side of the body, and the right side of the brain receives messages from the left side of the body. The movements of your right foot are controlled by the left side of your brain, while those of your left foot are controlled by your right brain. Nerves that connect the two halves of the brain let the whole brain know what is going on in both halves of the body.

If something happens to interrupt the flow of messages from the brain to the feet, they will become paralyzed, unable to move. A cutoff of sensory messages to the brain will make the feet feel numb, without their normal senses of touch, temperature, and pain. Similar effects may occur if the spinal cord is damaged, preventing the flow of messages to and from the feet. Damage to particular nerves can result in a partial paralysis or loss of sensation. In polio victims, the nerves that stimulate the *tibialis anterior* muscle are often damaged. This is a muscle in the front part of the lower leg that makes the foot bend upward at the ankle. The polio victim's foot tends to drag along, with the toes hanging downward because the muscle to lift them is no longer working.

Oddly enough, people who have had a foot amputated may still "feel" the foot as if it were still there. These "phantom" sensations are the result of stimulation of the ends of the nerves in the stump. Scientists are working on ways to use these still working nerves to develop "bionic" artificial limbs for amputees. Such artificial limbs could send the nerves messages very much like the sensory feedback from a real foot, and their movements would be guided by messages from the person's own motor nerves.

Recently a fad called firewalking has been making the news. People walk barefoot over hot coals without feeling any pain or getting burned. The sponsors of these events, selling expensive "self-improvement" programs, claim that their training helps people to walk through fire unharmed by using the power of their minds. But studies have shown that people without the expensive training can firewalk safely, too; and some people who try it are seriously burned even with the training. Part of the trick does indeed involve the mind. Firewalkers use various devices like repeating a soothing phrase over and over to distract themselves, so that they will not be conscious of the pain. Messages are sent from pain receptors in the soles of the feet, but the brain does not pay attention to them. (This kind of effect can happen in everyday life, too. Athletes injured during a sports event, for example, may be so absorbed that they do not even realize they are hurt until after the game is over.) The secret of getting across the hot coals unburned lies in principles of physics rather than in mysterious mental powers. The embers in a bed of hot coals are light and fluffy, and they do not conduct heat very well. They may seem very hot, but they do not contain enough heat energy to burn—as long as a person walks across them fast enough.

Skin, muscles, bones, and nerves—these are all living tissues that need continual supplies of energy and food to power their activities and repair damage. The food and oxygen that living cells need are carried by the blood, which flows through tubelike blood vessels. *Arteries* are blood vessels that carry blood away from the heart to the body. They branch and rebranch into smaller and smaller tubes, finally forming *capillaries*, which are tubes so tiny you need a microscope to see them. The capillaries have very thin walls. Oxy-

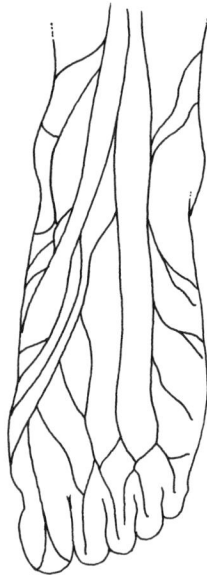 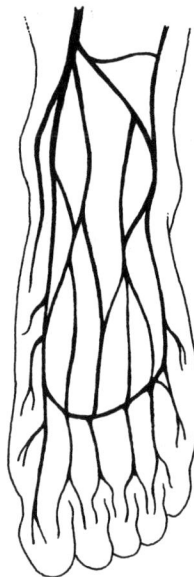 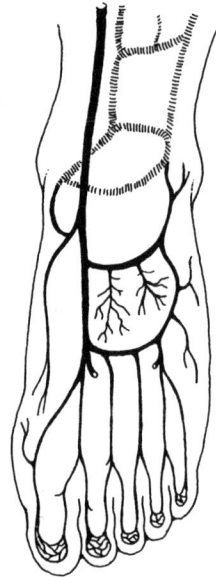

LYMPHATICS   VEINS   ARTERIES

gen and food substances pass out of them into the cells, and carbon dioxide and other waste products pass out of the cells into the capillaries. The capillaries join to form larger and larger tubes, eventually producing *veins,* blood vessels that carry blood back to the heart.

The oxygen-rich blood that the arteries carry to the body is bright red. When you look at your foot you can't see any arteries because they are buried deep inside the tissues. But you can see the paths of some of the veins that carry blood back from your foot. They appear as blue lines in the skin. Veins appear blue because the blood they carry is darker than the bright red arterial blood.

The heart is a muscular pump, which pumps blood forcefully out into the arteries. Arteries are rather thick-walled, and rhythmic contractions of their muscular walls help to send the blood speeding along. But when the blood gets to the capillaries it slows down. And the walls of the capillaries are so thin that some of the watery fluid from the blood leaks out into the tissues. Various chemicals are carried out too, but the red blood cells are too large to slip out through the leaky capillary walls. So the fluid that leaks into the tissues does not have the red color of blood. This pale, watery fluid is called *lymph*. Gradually it collects in tiny *lymph capillaries,* which join together into larger tubes called *lymphatics*. These are very much like veins, but they carry lymph instead of blood. They drain into two large *lymphatic ducts,* which eventually empty into the heart.

In most of the body, circulation works very effectively. Blood is carried from the heart through arteries to the capillaries that feed the body cells. The blood is returned to the heart by the veins, and meanwhile any fluid that has leaked out of the capillaries is returned by lymphatics. But both the veins and the lymphatics have much thinner walls than the arteries, and their walls are not muscular. They are equipped with special valves to keep the blood or lymph from flowing backward, but they don't have any pumping action to push it along. In the feet, this arrangement creates special problems. When a person is standing, the feet are the lowest part of the body, far lower than the heart. The body must work against the force of gravity to send the blood back up to the heart. During normal activities, the contractions of the leg muscles press on the veins and lymphatics, creating a pumping action that helps to re-

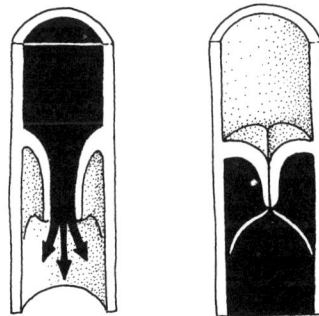

OPEN   CLOSED

turn the blood and lymph. Pressure changes associated with breathing also help. If you stand or sit perfectly still, though, there is not enough muscle action to be effective. Veins in the feet and lower legs expand as blood pools in them, and the fluid that leaks out of the capillaries accumulates in the tissues. The feet and ankles begin to swell. Meanwhile, not enough blood is being returned to the heart to be pumped out again to feed the body. The brain may not get enough blood to keep up its supply of oxygen and sugar, and you may start to feel dizzy and faint.

Some people really do faint after standing very still for a long time. That is what happens to some soldiers on parade when they fall down suddenly after standing at attention. Fainting quickly solves the circulation problem: As soon as the person is lying down flat, blood and lymph will be much more easily returned to the heart, and soon the brain will again be receiving all the energy materials it needs. Of course, most people don't faint, even when their ankles swell. If you have to stand for a long time, you can keep the blood flowing back normally by tensing and relaxing your leg muscles. People who sway or walk around when they are giving a speech are unconsciously keeping their circulation going. The main problem caused by pooling of fluids in the tissues of the feet during sitting is discomfort: Shoes fit tighter and may press on the swollen feet. (The situation may also be embarrassing, if you slip off your shoes to ease the pressure and can't get them back on.)

In addition to supplying oxygen and food to the body cells, the blood also acts as one of the body's main means of regulating its temperature. The blood that flows in capillaries close to the surface of the skin radiates excess heat out into the air. Normally your feet

46

feel comfortably warm as a result of the heat carried in these capillaries. But when you go into a cold place, the body switches on its heat-conserving system. Some of the blood vessels feeding the capillaries in the hands and feet close down and send the blood back toward the heart. That way the amount of heat lost by radiation through the skin is decreased. Even though the hands and feet are cold, the rest of the body—including important organs like the brain—is kept warm. In people suffering from a condition called *Raynaud's syndrome,* the body's temperature-control switches overwork. When the temperature outside the body is cold, so much of the circulation to the hands and feet is cut off that they become very cold and pale. Tissues may even be damaged, for lack of nourishing blood. In some people Raynaud's syndrome is part of a general body disease that affects the connective tissues. But it can also occur in young, otherwise healthy people. Not only cold but also strong emotions may trigger the attacks.

Speaking of cold feet: Exposure to extreme cold or cold wind may cause a very serious problem called *frostbite.* The blood and fluid in the tissues literally freeze, cutting off the circulation. The toes, fingers, ears, and tip of the nose are usually the first parts of the body to be affected. The frostbitten areas turn pale, and if they are not warmed soon, tissue may be destroyed. It used to be thought that the best thing to do for someone with frostbite was to rub the frozen parts with snow. But rubbing can break down the tissues. Instead, the frostbitten parts should be placed in warm water or wrapped in warm blankets. It's better to avoid frostbite by not staying outside in very cold weather for long periods and by dressing in warm clothes that are not too tight.

47

∘ 4 ∘

Feet in Action

Did you know that the muscles of your body are working hard when you are standing still? They must struggle against the pull of gravity, which would tend to make you collapse in a heap like a rag doll if there were nothing to oppose it. What's more, your muscles not only have to keep you up; they have to keep you up straight. Otherwise you would topple over onto your nose or the back of your head.

Like the inner framework of the feet, the skeleton that forms the inner framework of the rest of the body is not one solid, rigid structure. Instead it is made up of a series of bones, jointed together into a long curving cylinder, the *spinal column.* The spine can be flexible when you need to bend over, but the muscles, tendons, and ligaments attached to it can lock it into a rigid center post when you need to stand up straight. This apparent rigidity is the result of dozens of continuing adjustments, as groups of muscles play tug-of-war with other muscles to place each body part in just the right place. All these muscle actions are carefully coordinated by messages from the brain. The coordination centers in the brain receive a continual flow of information: from sense receptors in the soles of the feet and the joints of the feet and legs; from the eyes, to let the brain know whether things look right-side-up or tipped over; and from special balance organs inside the ears, where a combination of sloshing fluids, tiny stones, and sensitive hairs responds to a change of position in any direction. (If you get dizzy on a merry-go-round, it is because the balance organs in the inner ears can't keep up with the constant changes.)

The aim of all that muscle work is to keep your *center of gravity* firmly positioned above your feet. (Your body, like any other solid, behaves as though all its weight were concentrated at one imaginary point, the center of gravity. It is usually, but not always, somewhere around the middle part of the body.) Meanwhile, your feet are rigidly locked into what foot doctors call the *neutral position.* This is the most efficient position for holding up the body. In the neutral position a normal foot is not completely flattened under the weight of the body: The weight is borne by the ball of the foot and the heel, and the middle part is raised in an arch. The height of the arch differs greatly among individuals but this variation is quite normal and healthy.

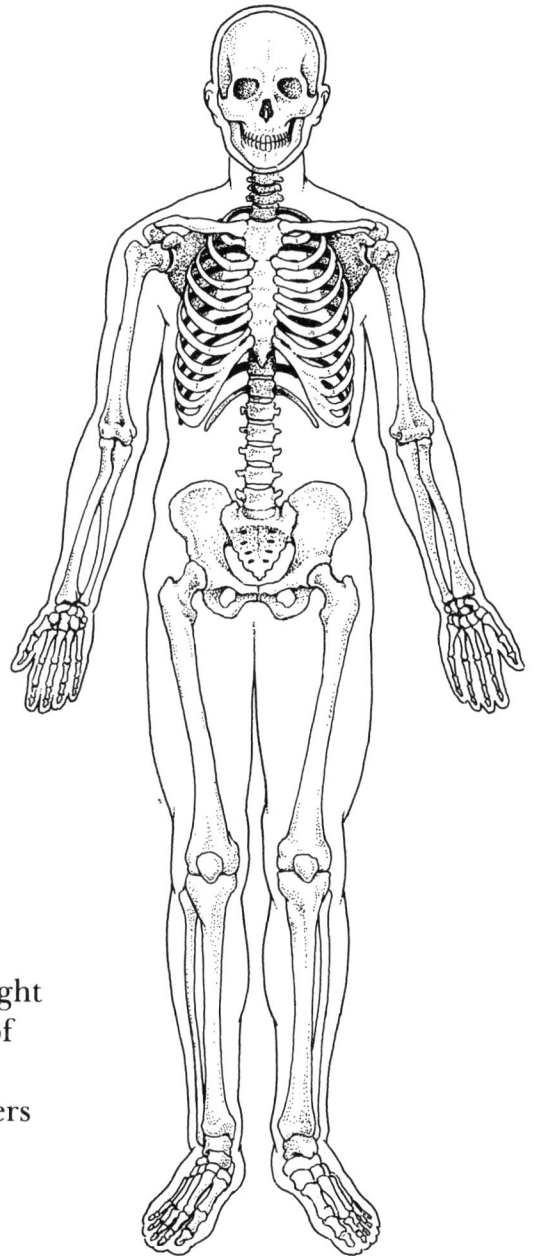

Wearing high heels shifts a person's center of gravity forward. To avoid falling over, the tendency is to pull the upper part of the body backward, compensating for the extra weight in front. The result is a "swayback" posture, which can produce backaches and other ailments as the muscles overwork to keep the body in balance. Another result of wearing high heels is a gradual shortening of the Achilles tendon. A person used to high heels, who tries to switch to low heels, suffers from aching calf muscles because of the unaccustomed stretching of the tendon. Doctors recommend that shoes have heels no higher than an inch and a half. If higher heels are worn, switching to lower heels for part of the day helps to keep the gastrocnemius muscle in good condition.

If maintaining good posture while standing still sounds like a lot of hard work, imagine what the muscles have to do when the body is moving around! Walking up stairs, for example, requires the coordinated work of about three hundred different muscles. Each time you take a step, your center of gravity shifts, and your brain and muscles have to work out a whole new combination of efforts to keep you upright.

Insects have some advantages over us in ease of getting around. They move their six legs in groups of three, one on one side and two on the other. That way, the insect's body is always firmly supported by a stable tripod of legs, and its center of gravity stays

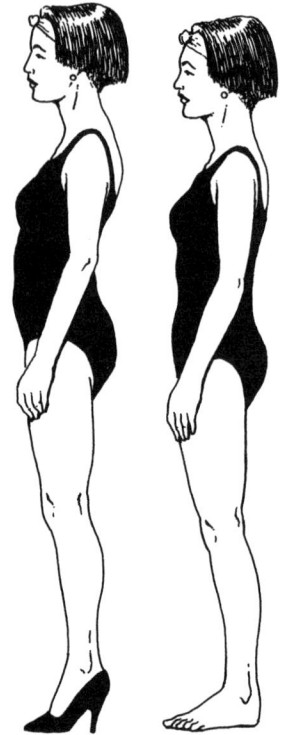

nicely balanced. Four-legged animals also have it easier than we do. In walking, they pick up one foot at a time, leaving a tripod of legs firmly planted on the ground. Even when a four-legged animal runs, it still has two feet on the ground at all times. An elephant can't run at all. Its weight is too heavy to be supported on just two legs. With three feet on the ground at all times, an elephant that seems to be running is really only walking very fast.

For bipeds like us humans, moving around is a real balancing act. Continual adjustments of the body muscles, coordinated by the brain, are needed to compensate for the continually shifting center of gravity. It is mainly the cerebellum that coordinates our movements, with only rare assistance from the cerebrum. Once you learn how to walk and run, all the complicated movements involved become so automatic that you do not have to think about them consciously.

LOCOMOTION

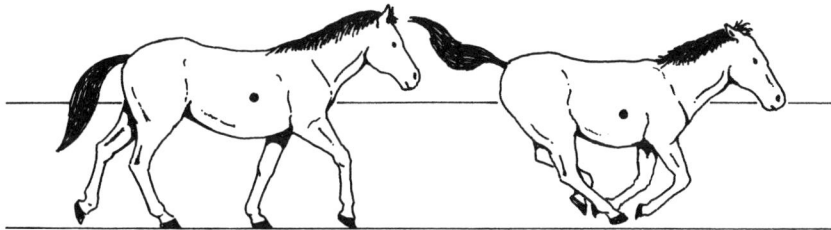

quadruped

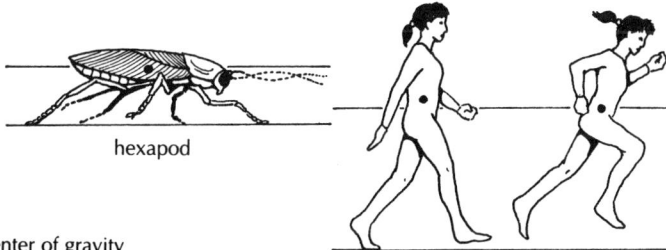

hexapod

● = center of gravity

biped

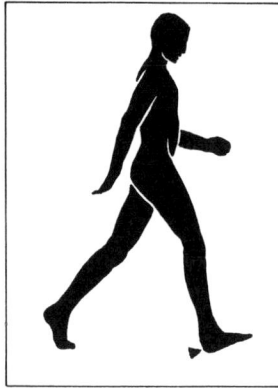

1. Heel hits first.   *2. Weight on mid-foot.*   *3. Weight transfers to ball.*

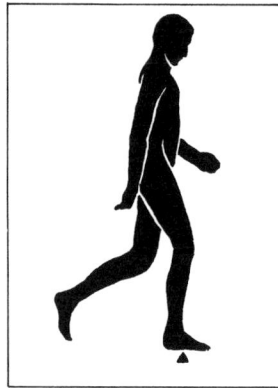

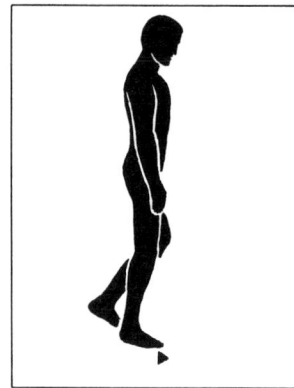

What is the difference between walking and running? You are probably tempted to say it is a matter of speed: A person running goes much faster than one who is walking. But racewalkers cover the ground at a pace of five miles an hour—considerably below the fifteen miles an hour of an Olympic miler, but a lot faster than the normal strolling pace of two or three miles an hour. The real difference between walking and running is the number of feet on the ground. In walking, there is one foot on the ground at all times, while in running both feet are off the ground during a portion of every stride.

When you take a step, strong contractions in the muscles of the thigh swing one of your legs forward. Muscles of the lower leg keep the foot partly extended, ready for contact with the ground. Meanwhile, in the leg that is still on the ground supporting your body, contractions of the calf muscles, the gastrocnemius and soleus, raise you on tiptoe and then push off. The leg that was swinging

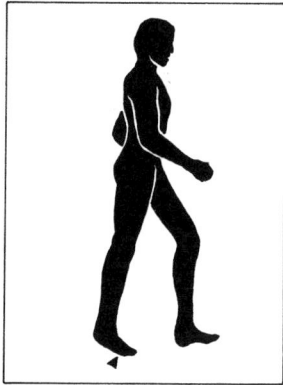

| 4. Full weight on ball and toes. | 5. Toes push off. | 6. Whole foot off ground. |

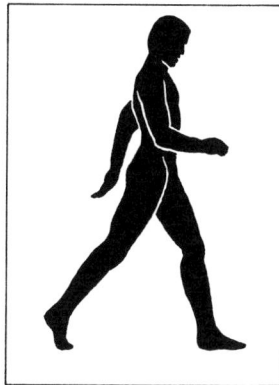

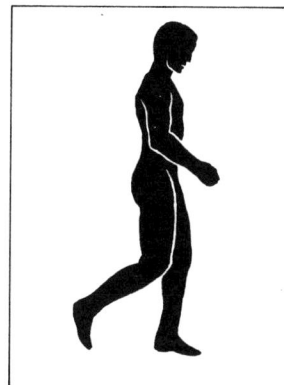

forward meets the ground heel first. The fleshy pad on the bottom of the heel helps cushion the first shock of contact, and the shock is gradually transmitted down the arch to the ball of the foot as the front of your foot makes contact. Sense receptors give a continuous flow of feedback to the brain about the kind of surface you have stepped on, and the foot adapts automatically to it. Then contractions of the foot and leg muscles lock it firmly in place, forming a stable platform from which to launch the next step.

Humans have a manner of walking that scientists refer to as *plantigrade,* which means that we walk on the soles of our feet. Some members of the animal kingdom share this plantigrade walk. Our monkey and ape relatives walk flat on the soles of their feet. (Actually, monkeys scamper about plantigrade on four foot-hands.) Bear footprints look very similar to those of a human (a rather flatfooted human) because they, too, have a plantigrade walk. Some of the reports of mysterious humanlike "abominable snowmen" glimpsed

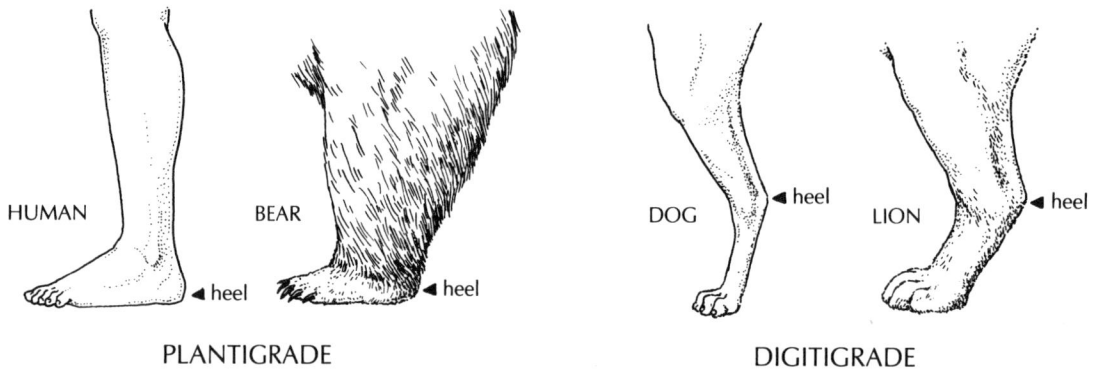

HUMAN   BEAR   DOG   LION

◄ heel   ◄ heel   ◄ heel   ◄ heel

PLANTIGRADE   DIGITIGRADE

in out-of-the-way places are based on bear prints and sightings of bears walking on their hind legs.

When an animal (or a person) switches from a walk to a fast run, there is a natural tendency to go up onto the toes. Animals that specialize in speed go around on their toes full time. What we think of as the "foot" of a cat or dog is actually just the ball of the foot, plus the toes. Its "knees" seem to be bent at the wrong angle because they aren't really knees at all; they are ankles. This kind of walk is called *digitigrade*. The hoofed mammals, which are among nature's speediest, take toe-walking one step further: They walk on their toenails. The tough hooves at the bottom of a horse's or antelope's feet are actually modified nails. Fossils of these animals' ancestors suggest that all the hoofed mammals started out with the standard five toes, but some of them gradually lost toes in the long chain of generations. Elephants still have the original five toes— that much weight needs a broad platform to support it. Hippos and pigs have four toes, but the pig puts all its weight on the two big middle toes. The two outer toes are little things, too high up on the leg to touch the ground. The rhinoceros walks on three toenails, with one big middle toe and two small ones on the sides. The foot

54

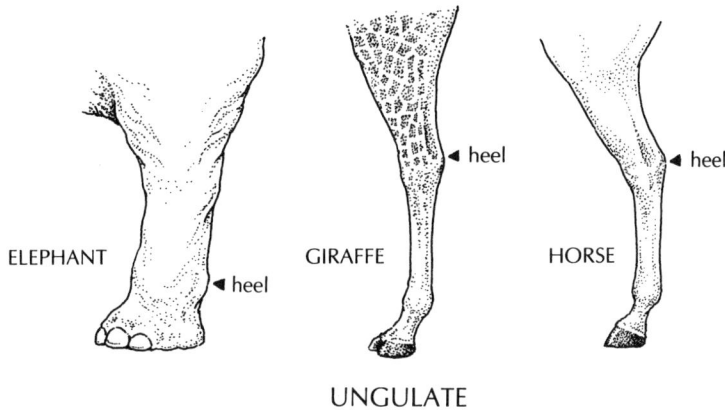

ELEPHANT   ◄ heel

◄ heel

GIRAFFE   ◄ heel

HORSE   ◄ heel

UNGULATE

of the giraffe is streamlined down to two toes, and the horse's hoof is just a single broad toenail. The animals that walk on their toenails are called *ungulates*. Humans can walk on tiptoes, but it is more difficult to keep your balance this way than when you use the whole foot to support you. A ballerina must put in long hours of practice to be able to support herself on a single big toe in a pirouette, and even then she could not do it without the bracing of a specially designed shoe.

Some animals use jumping or leaping to cover ground quickly or to break away suddenly to escape from an enemy. The best leapers in the animal kingdom belong to a variety of groups, from insects to mammals, but they all have some characteristics in common. They all have one pair of legs (usually the hind legs) that are larger and stronger than the others, and these legs are equipped with powerful sets of muscles that work to launch the animal's body with a vigorous push against the solid surface. If you look at yourself in the mirror, you'll notice that you seem to fit that description fairly well. How do humans compare to the best jumpers in the animal world? Well, a human champion broad jumper can leap about eleven feet, which is better than the foot or so that a flea can

length of leap   relative distance compared to length of animal

flea: 1'   200x

frog: 17'   30x

kangaroo: 26'   5x

human: 11'   2x

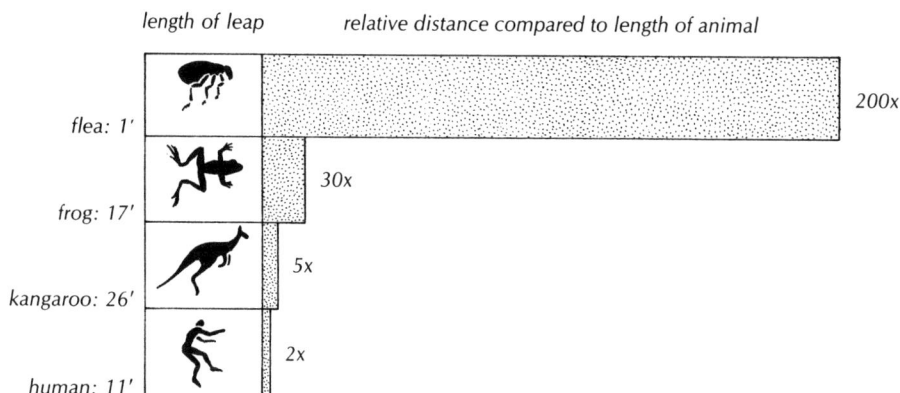

manage. But the longest recorded leap by a frog was over seventeen feet, and a kangaroo can cover twenty-six feet in one jump. Looking at the question in another way, a human can jump a distance of about two times his or her height, a kangaroo can leap five times its height, a frog as much as thirty times its height, and the tiny flea can leap over a distance about *two hundred times* the length of its body.

Getting around in the water—swimming—presents some different problems. Water has buoyancy: It helps to hold your body up, so you do not have to work so hard against gravity. But water presents more resistance to body movements than air does, though not as much as solid ground, against which the feet push in walking and running. The arms are important in swimming, knifing through the water and pushing it aside like paddles. But the feet are important, too. Kicking provides a substantial part of the force that propels you through the water.

These days people are very fitness minded, and many people take part in regular exercises to keep their bodies in tone. Active

56

exercises that have a toning effect on the heart and lungs are especially good for maintaining and improving health. Such exercises are called *aerobic exercises,* because they increase the body's ability to use oxygen from the air efficiently.

Walking is one of the best exercises for strengthening the heart and lungs, and it is the best one to start with for people who are out of shape. Walking doesn't require any expensive equipment, and you can walk anywhere, any time. By adjusting the amount of time they spend walking and the pace, people in a wide range of physical conditions can get healthy exercise. You can tell whether an exercise is strenuous enough to build heart and lung strength by taking your pulse. It should be higher than usual but should fall within a "target zone" that varies with age. For a ten-year-old, the pulse rate during aerobic exercise should be between 150 and 180 beats per minute. The target range falls gradually, to 140 to 170 for a twenty-year-old, 120 to 145 for a fifty-year-old, and about 105 to 125 for a seventy-year-old. For many people, walking at a pace of a mile in about 15 or 20 minutes is enough to bring their pulse rate up into the target zone. A very brisk walking pace would cover a mile in about 12 minutes. Counting another way, a pace of about 130 to 140 steps per minute can provide good exercise.

As you get into better condition, though, ordinary walking may

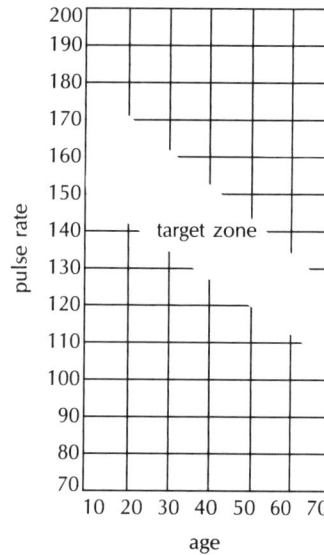

57

not be enough to raise your pulse into the target zone. Then you need to go to the special techniques of racewalking or switch to jogging.

Racewalking is an exercise sport that has been gaining in popularity. It is more than just walking at a very fast pace; it is a whole new way of walking, involving swinging movements of the hips and rhythmic movements of the arms and upper body. The result is that the upper body stays level (in regular walking or in jogging, the whole body bobs up and down with each step), and the smooth technique and longer stride mean that the racewalker can cover more ground faster than an ordinary walker and does not tire as quickly as a runner. The feet—and the spine—are spared the jolts that a runner's steps produce, and injuries are very rare.

Jogging is a slow run. Your foot hits the ground with the heel first, as in walking (when you sprint, your toe comes down first), but the legs and arms move faster and more rhythmically than in walking. Special jogging shoes are needed to cushion the ankles, knees, hips, and back against the jolts that occur when the feet strike the ground. (Racewalking, on the other hand, is less jarring on the body. It is becoming popular among former joggers with injuries that prevent them from running.) Before walking or jogging, you should do some exercises to stretch the muscles of your lower back and the backs of your legs. After jogging it is best to have a "cooling down" period of walking around slowly, rather than stopping short and flopping down.

For aerobic exercise to benefit the heart and lungs, your pulse rate should be in the target zone for at least 20 to 30 minutes at a time, and you should exercise at least three times a week. According to the experts, there's not much extra benefit from exercising every day, and—especially when you are first starting an exercise program—a day off between exercise sessions gives the muscles a chance to recover and helps to prevent strains. There is an easy test to determine whether you are exercising too hard for your body: You should have enough energy (and breath) left over to hold a conversation while you walk or run. If you can't talk while you walk, you're going too fast.

Swimming and bicycling are also good aerobic exercises. Like walking and running, they involve continuous rhythmic movements that build stamina. Sports like tennis or basketball are fun, but they are "start-and-stop" exercises that do not do as much to strengthen the heart and lungs. Sudden stops, starts, and twisting movements involved in these sports can also put stress on muscles and joints and result in injuries.

Running, jumping, and other forms of foot action are important parts of sports such as tennis, basketball, and baseball. But there are several popular sports in which the feet themselves are used as tools for moving a ball around. Actually, the term "football" can mean different things, depending on where you live. In most countries of the world it refers to the game that Americans call soccer. In Great Britain, there is also the sport of rugby football. The kind of football played in the United States is still another kind of game. All three sports, American-style football, soccer, and rugby, are team sports played on a rectangular field, in which one team tries to move a ball past the goal line or through the goal posts of the opposing team. The rules of the games differ quite a bit, and so do the balls used: A soccer ball, for example, is a large round inflated ball with a leather cover, while a football is smaller and sort of egg-shaped, with pointed ends and so is the ball used in rugby. One

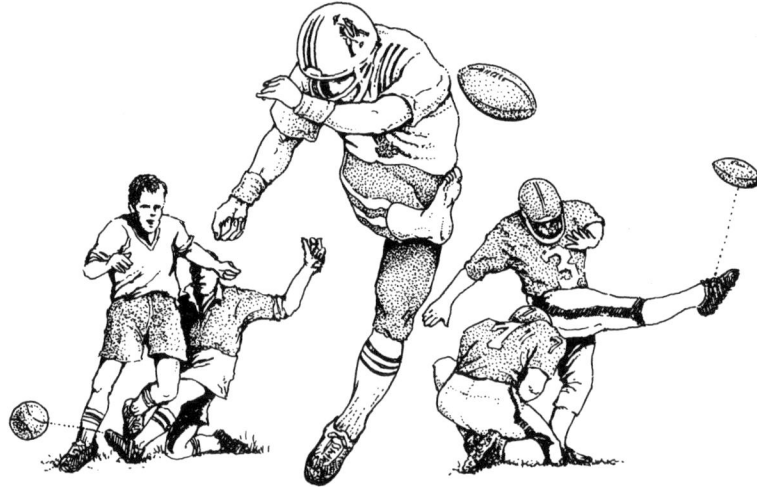

thing football, soccer, and rugby all have in common is the use of kicking with the feet to move the ball around.

In walking, running, and most other activities involving movement from one place to another, the feet serve as dynamic supports, which hold up the body and propel it along. In kicking, the aim is different: Instead of moving the body, the kicking foot is using body energy to move something else, such as a ball. One foot stays on the ground to provide support and balance, while the other leg is swung like a pendulum, hits the ball with a solid impact, and transfers the energy of the swing to it, sending it flying off into the air.

Traditionally, the kicking techniques used in American-style football and in soccer are quite different. The football kicker uses either a place kick (in which a teammate holds the ball balanced on its point on the ground or on a small tee) or a drop kick. The kicker's toe contacts the ball first, and then the foot smoothly molds to the contour of the ball, which fits into the curve of the instep as the momentum of the swing sends it flying away. Soccer players, on the other hand, typically kick the ball with the instep, with the inner or outer side of the foot, or with the heel. The instep is the most effective kick, since the soccer player can best control the length, the accuracy, and the power of the kick. In any case, the follow-through (the continuing swing of the kicking leg after it meets the ball) is very important in directing the flight of the ball. Recently a number of former soccer players have become specialized kickers for football teams and have brought the instep kick along with them. One NFL kicking star, Tony Franklin of the Philadelphia Eagles, does his kicking barefoot. After a game, his instep is red and sore.

With the emphasis on exercise and fitness, the science of *biomechanics* has become an active field of research. Sports physicians and physiologists study the movements and forces involved in walking, running, and other activities. Computers that can simulate body movements and predict how muscles and bones will react in new situations are providing a powerful new research tool. There have already been some practical applications from such studies. Biomechanics has made it possible to design better running shoes, which provide more effective cushioning and support. Studies at Harvard University even yielded a special "tuned" track for the college track team. The track has a special surface of polyethylene, which stores some of the energy from a runner's step and returns it to his foot when he takes the next stride. The first year the new track was open, the Harvard team increased their speeds by an average of 3 percent. Even better, the springier track surface allowed the runners to train harder without risking muscle strains and other injuries.

·5·

Foot Fitness

The feet of a young man from Michigan were in the news recently. Eighteen-year-old Allen Pepke had wanted to join the Army, but recruiters turned him down because of a foot problem. Determined to prove he was fit to serve in spite of his problem, Pepke set off on a hike—all the way from his home in Michigan to the nation's capital, Washington, D.C. He traveled most of the way on foot, and government officials were so impressed that the Army signed him up after all, and the Governor of Michigan treated him to a tour of Washington as his guest.

Most foot problems don't make the news, but they are important in the lives of many people. They are also more common than they used to be, now that many more people are taking part in activities like jogging and aerobic dancing, which put extra stresses on the feet. A recent survey of more than a thousand students and instructors in aerobic dance classes, for example, showed that nearly half of them had been injured during the exercises. Injuries are probably just as common among joggers. This is not surprising, considering that each running step concentrates three to four times the weight of the body on the foot. Even people who do not exercise regularly can suffer from foot problems. These may be due to structural defects in the feet that put unnatural stresses on the bones or muscles. Poorly fitting or badly designed footwear can cause problems, and feet can also suffer from infections such as athlete's foot and plantar warts.

A doctor who specializes in foot problems is called a *podiatrist.* Podiatrists are licensed by the state and must have completed a program of education and training comparable to those of other doctors. First a minimum of three (or preferably four) years of college premedical courses are needed. Then comes a four-year program at a college of podiatric medicine. (There are only six of them in the United States.) During the first two years the student takes the same sort of basic science courses as other medical and dental students, in subjects such as anatomy, physiology, biochemistry, microbiology, pharmacology, and pathology, along with specialized courses in podiatric medicine and surgery. The last two years provide practical experience in patient care. About two thirds of the graduates from podiatric colleges take one to three years of residency in a hospital, where they gain additional experience in treating emergency cases and more specialized problems such as those of children, the elderly, or athletes. In most states practicing podiatrists must also take continuing courses on the latest advances in their field in order to renew their licenses.

How do you know when you have a foot problem that needs the attention of a podiatrist? Itchy rashes that won't go away; swollen or hardened painful areas on the toes or other parts of the feet; pains in the foot muscles that keep recurring even though there may not be any obvious reason for them—these are all clear signs that something is wrong. (Foot problems may also cause aches and pains in other parts of the body, such as the legs and back, as the other muscles overwork to compensate.) But are there warning signs that can alert you to developing foot problems before they become serious?

Each person has his or her own individual way of standing and walking, which may not match the ideal. One person's toes may turn in; another may tend to toe out in standing and walking. A person's ankles may roll inward (a condition called *pronation*) or out toward the sides of the feet *(supination)*. Some people's legs do not form the normal straight lines when they stand at ease: They may be *knock-kneed* (the feet are apart while the knees are touching) or *bowlegged* (when the feet are together there is a space between the knees). The arch of the foot may be higher or lower than normal; or the foot may flatten out completely during standing *(flat feet)*. Your shoes can provide clues to how you stand and walk. If the soles and heels are wearing evenly, then you probably have well-formed, well-balanced feet. But shoes whose soles are worn down more on the outside, or on the inside, or perhaps in one particular

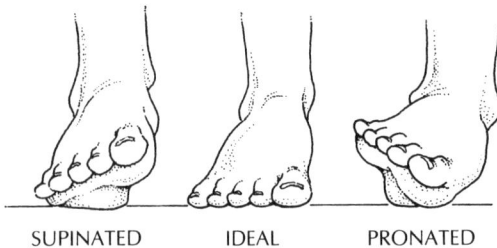

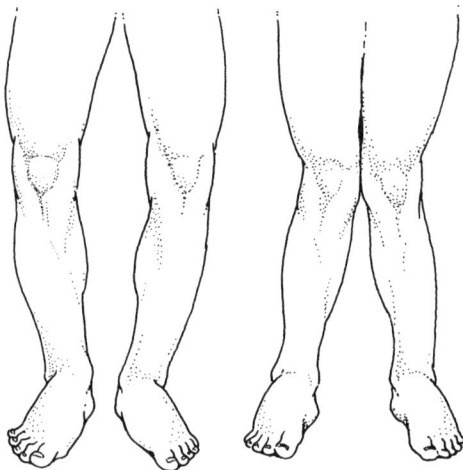

SUPINATED   IDEAL   PRONATED

BOWLEGS   KNOCK KNEES

spot on the heel point to foot problems. So do shoes whose uppers are bent and twisted out of shape, or have lumpy bulges, or tend to get scuffed in one spot.

Pronation and supination are part of the normal walking stride. When you first put your foot down in a step, it pronates slightly as the foot adapts to the walking surface and

ABNORMAL FLAT FEET

the bones of the arch take up the shock of contact. Then the arch rises again and the foot rolls upward and outward as it locks into place, ready to support the weight of the body and push off for another step. But if the foot is pronated all the time, it must support the body when it is not in its strongest position. The foot and leg muscles are called upon to do extra work, which may strain them; and unnatural stresses are placed on the bones, which may lead to bone and joint problems. Other variations from the normal foot structure can also lead to the development of foot ailments.

Podiatrists differ in their opinions on what role shoes play in the development of foot problems. Sometimes badly fitting shoes seem obviously to be at fault; yet such disorders as bunions have also been observed among people who go barefoot all the time. Probably foot problems are the result of a combination of factors: structural defects, which are often hereditary, and the pressures and stresses exerted by the wrong kind of shoes, which can eventually damage even healthy feet but affect feet with an unstable structure far more quickly. We have already mentioned some of the problems high heels can cause. Another bad shoe design, which unfortunately is often considered very stylish, is the pointed-toe shoe. Its

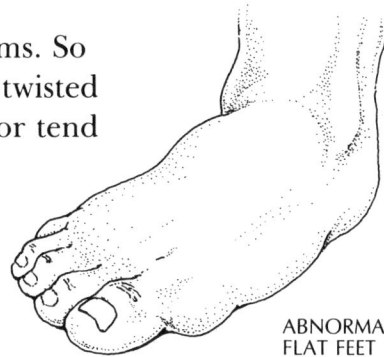

shape doesn't look at all like that of a real human foot: To fit into it comfortably, you'd have to have your big toe in the middle and smaller toes on the ends. When you try to fit a real foot into a pointed shoe, the inside of the shoe may press on your toes unless you get a larger size. (But many people—women, especially—tend to buy the smallest shoes they can possibly tolerate, because they think small feet look more attractive.)

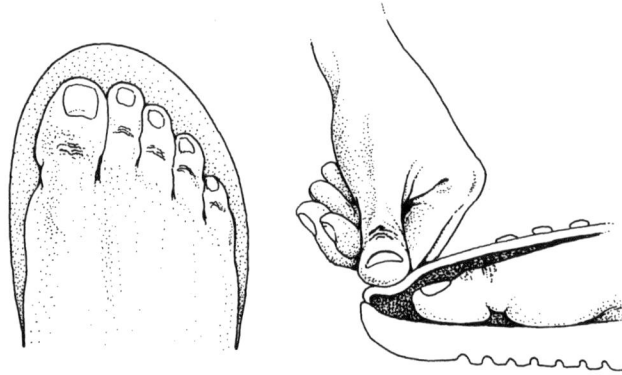

When you are getting a new pair of shoes, it is best to have them fitted near the end of the day, when your feet have spread out a bit from standing and walking. Make sure the shoe is not pressing on your toes or the sides of your feet. Don't buy shoes that are a little tight, figuring that you will "break them in"; new shoes should feel just as comfortable as your old shoes, from the very beginning. If your feet are still growing, make sure there is plenty of extra room in front. You should be able to wiggle your toes inside the shoes, and if someone presses down on the front of the shoe, there should be a full thumb's width of space in front of your big toe. Growing children need to get new shoes as often as every three months.

Buying shoes to wear for athletic activities presents special problems. There is no one all-purpose shoe that is good for every activity. Jogging, tennis, basketball, aerobic dancing—all have their own special requirements. Shoes for running need plenty of shock-absorbing cushioning on the soles. But the broad, flared heels on running shoes don't provide the proper support for the twisting motions of aerobic dancing and can result in ankle sprains. The stop-and-start, back-and-forth movements on a basketball court require a different kind of sole surface from the one-direction movements in running.

Foot doctors used to believe that any deviations from "normal" foot structure in young children had to be treated early in order to avoid more serious problems in later life, and they prescribed heavy orthopedic shoes and various other devices such as braces to be worn at night. Now doctors realize that some conditions that

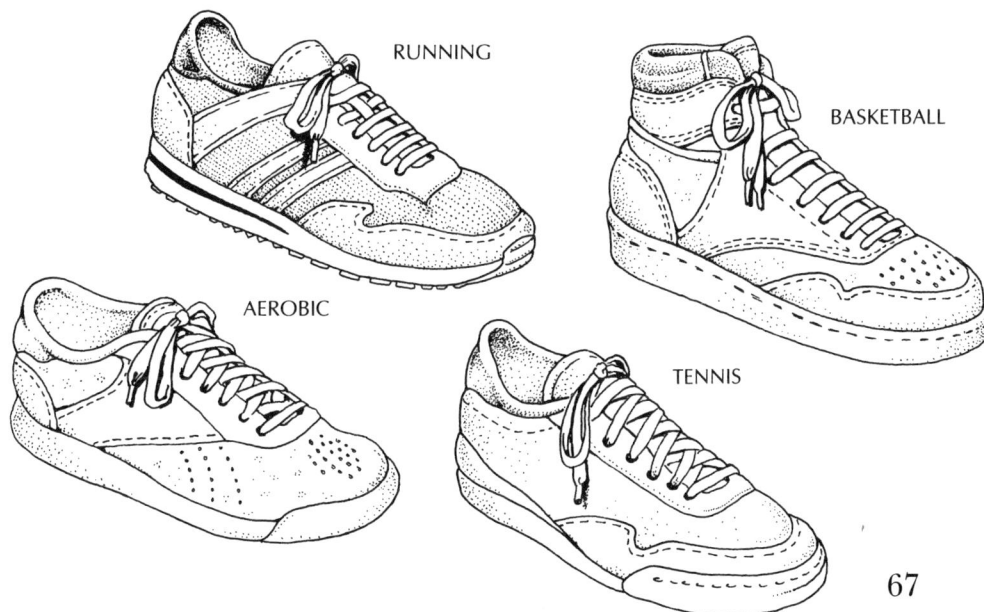

RUNNING

BASKETBALL

AEROBIC

TENNIS

67

used to be thought to be "defects" are actually part of the normal process of development. The "flat" feet of babies and young children usually reveal normal arches after the fat pads that hid them are lost. Feet that tend to toe in or out may straighten out by themselves by the age of eight or ten months. Bowlegs are normal in babies and toddlers up to the age of about two; then they pass through a knock-kneed phase, which ends at the age of five or six. If any of these conditions persist past the age when they normally disappear, they may have to be treated with casts, braces, special shoes, or even surgery.

Older children and adults with a variety of foot problems are helped by specially designed inserts that can be transferred from one pair of shoes to another. These inserts may be as simple as a felt or foam-rubber heel pad or an arch support. Or the podiatrist may make plaster molds of the person's feet and design custom-made *orthotics*. These shoe inserts provide support and pressure in just the right places to correct faulty alignments and bring the foot into a more efficient neutral position. Properly designed orthotics can be a great help not only in athletic activities but also in daily life, especially for people who must stand or walk a lot.

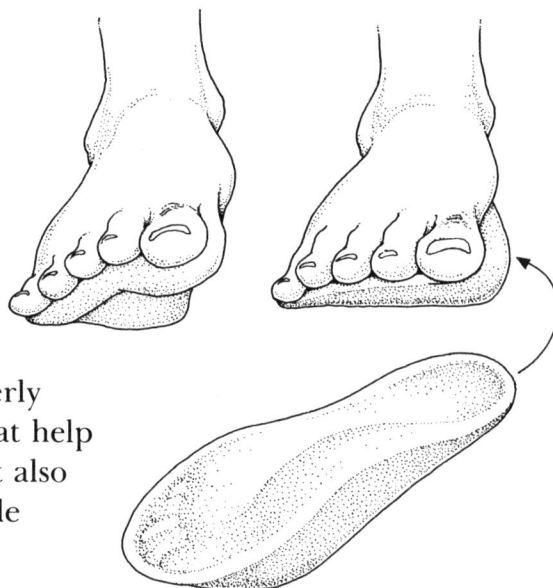

Following is a brief rundown of some common foot problems. More detailed information on these and other conditions, along with effective ways of treating them, can be found in the books listed at the end of the chapter.

Traumatic injuries. Feet can be injured in accidents, just like other parts of the body. Their skin may be cut or burned or bruised. If you have a deep cut, especially a puncture wound, be sure that your tetanus protection is up to date. If you have not had an immunization within ten years, get a booster shot. Accidents may also break or *fracture* the bones of the feet. (One of our daughters suffered a broken big toe when a frozen turkey slipped out of her hands and fell on it; stubbing the toe against something hard can also fracture the phalanges.)

Sudden twisting of an ankle can cause a *sprain,* which is a stretching and/or tearing of the ligaments that bind the bones of the joint together. The sprain may just be a minor pull, which will recover quickly. If you can walk on the foot without pain after it has had a few minutes to recover, then it is safe to go back to your activities. But if you can't put weight on it without pain, then the best first aid is a combination that sports-medicine specialists call *R.I.C.E.*— Rest, Ice, Compression, and Elevation. Resting the injured joint lets the natural healing processes take place. Ice should be applied within fifteen minutes of the injury and kept in place for periods of fifteen minutes at a time over the first few days. Ice helps to keep the injured joint from swelling and also helps to stimulate an increase in the blood supply as the body tries to warm up the injured part. Compression is applied in the form of an elastic bandage or tape strapping, which reduces swelling and limits the movement of the joint. Elevating the bottom of the mattress at night by placing some books under it raises the foot and lets gravity help to drain the excess fluids.

What is the difference between a sprain and a strain? A sprain is an injury to a joint, usually involving ligaments and tendons. A strain is an injury to a muscle, usually due to overuse. Muscles may recover from a strain within a couple of weeks if you do not reinjure them by going back to exercising too soon, but tears in ligaments may take even longer to heal than a bone fracture.

Pressure problems. Some chronic and painful foot problems can result from the foot's own efforts to protect itself. A *callus* is a thickening of the skin that occurs in response to too much pressure. Calluses typically form on the sole in the region of the ball of the foot, under the heads of the metatarsal bones. They may also occur on the toes or heel. Heel calluses may crack, especially when open-back shoes are worn, and then they may become infected. But if a callus is not causing pain and is not very thick, it is not a problem that needs special attention. You can help to keep it under control by rubbing it regularly with a pumice stone or sandpaper file.

Shoes don't cause calluses. (They actually help to prevent or control them by taking up some of the shocks of walking and running.) But poorly fitting shoes can contribute to the formation of *corns*. These are small areas of thickened skin, usually on the toes. The corn may have a hard, dense nucleus, which may lie over a point of maximum pressure, such as a pointed bone. Soft corns may form on the surfaces between toes. Corns hurt when they become inflamed or when they press on sensitive nerves. Trying to treat a corn yourself can be tricky and dangerous. Medicated pads

70

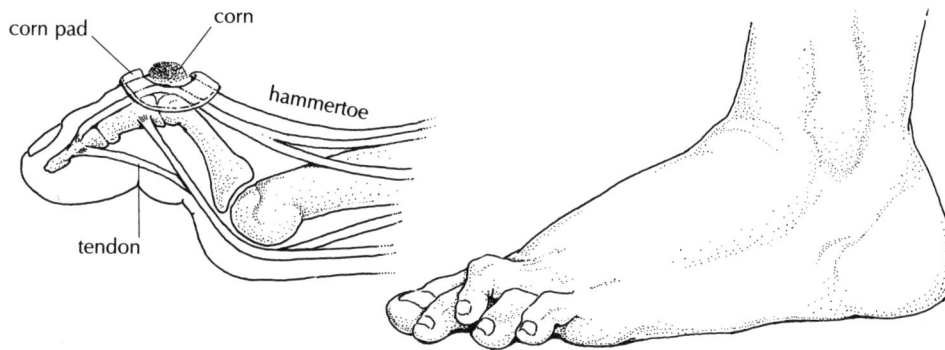

HAMMER THIRD TOE

sold in drugstores can cause chemical burns, and if you try to trim away the corn with a razor blade you may cut the living skin around it, causing bleeding and perhaps infection. A podiatrist can safely trim excess tissue from a corn, but that does not "cure" it. To get lasting relief you have to eliminate the cause of the excess pressure, perhaps by getting larger shoes or spot-stretching the ones you have. Circular foam or felt pads, which are placed on the healthy skin around the corn, can relieve the pressure and help healing. If a corn is the result of a structural defect, such as *hammertoe* (a condition in which a toe is pushed up with the knuckle raised), surgery may be needed to correct it.

A *bunion* is an unsightly and painful bump that forms on the big toe joint. The *bursa,* the tough fluid-filled sac that surrounds the joint, is inflamed, usually because of a structural problem. (Tight-fitting shoes can make the problem worse.) Warm foot soaks and

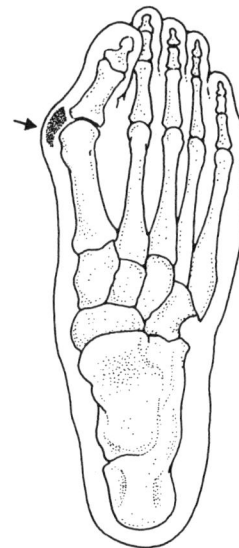

aspirin are helpful in relieving pain from bunions. Shoes with extra room in front can relieve some of the pressure and add to comfort. A custom-made bunion shield can also be effective. The condition can be corrected by surgery that not only removes the bump but realigns the bones so that the bunion will not form again.

A *blister* is an accumulation of fluid under the outer layer of skin. It forms when the inside of the shoe rubs against the skin or when the skin is caught between a tight shoe and the bones of the foot, which move during the normal foot movements. Blisters form most often on the back of the heel, on the toes, and on the ball of the foot. If a blister is small, it is best to just let it alone, meanwhile relieving the pressure by changing to looser shoes or surrounding the blister with a foam or felt pad with the middle cut out. If the blister is large, massage it with ice for about fifteen minutes (this acts as an anesthetic), wash it thoroughly and apply a disinfectant such as Merthiolate, and then make a few puncture holes carefully near one end of the blister with a sterilized needle. (A needle can be sterilized by passing it through a flame or dipping it in alcohol.) Then press gently on the blister to make the fluid ooze out through the holes. When it is completely drained, leave the top of the blister in place and cover the area with a Band-Aid or other clean dressing. The skin that was raised will protect the damaged tissues from infection and will reattach itself as the blister heals.

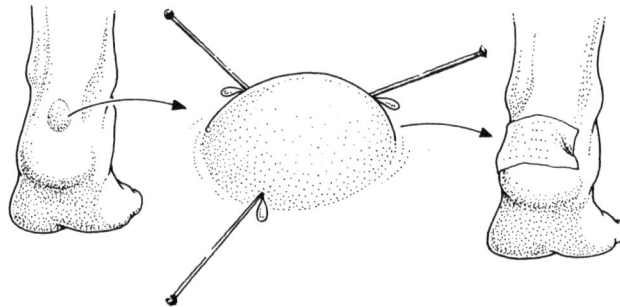

Ingrown toenails occur when the edge of the toenail curls under and digs into the surrounding skin. This painful condition is usually caused by cutting the toenails incorrectly, but tight shoes can contribute to the problem. The skin around the ingrown toenail may become callused, or bacteria may enter the cut and cause infections. The condition is treated by carefully cutting away the curved-under portion of the nail at the corner; it is safest to have this done by a podiatrist.

Heel spurs are extra growths of bone under the heel in response to strain at the point where the *plantar fascia,* the tough sheet of fibrous tissue that lies under the skin of the sole, is attached to the heel bone. The spur provides some extra bony support at a point of strain, and a person who has one may never be aware of it. But heel spurs can cause pain when the strain becomes too great and the bursa surrounding the spur becomes inflamed. Pain and inflammation can be reduced by using anti-inflammatory drugs such as cortisone derivatives. Padding the arch, strapping the foot, or using specially designed shock-absorbing heel cups or innersoles can relieve the strain on the heel. Joggers suffering from "runner's heel" can also get some relief by changing their running technique to shift more of the body weight onto the middle or front of the foot in each running step.

Infections. You don't have to be an athlete to suffer from *athlete's foot.* It is a fungus infection that causes itchy, peeling skin, especially between the toes. You may pick up the tiny fungus spores by walking barefoot in a shower room or some other place where an infected person has been walking. The athlete's foot fungus grows best in warm, moist surroundings. If you wear sneakers without

REGULAR TOENAIL

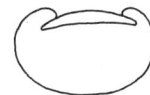

INGROWN TOENAIL

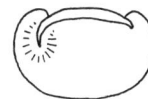

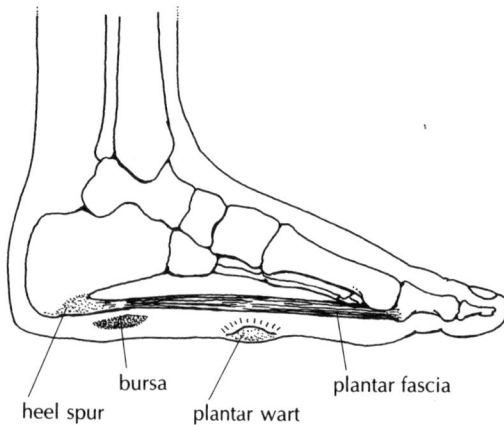

heel spur   bursa   plantar wart   plantar fascia

socks, you are providing the fungus with an ideal environment. The infection is treated with medicated powders or creams, but for lasting relief you also need to cut down on foot sweating by wearing well ventilated shoes and cotton or wool socks that soak up moisture and draw it away from the foot. Don't wear the same pair of shoes every day; give the shoes at least a day to rest and dry out.

A round hard lump of thickened skin on the sole of the foot may seem like a corn, and indeed it may be one. Corns sometimes form inside calluses, over a point of special pressure. But a lump on the bottom of the foot may be a *plantar wart*. Like the warts that grow on the hands and other places, plantar warts are caused by viruses that slip into a cut or sore, and they are very contagious. Instead of growing out into a rough, cauliflowerlike lump as warts on other parts of the body do, plantar warts are constantly subjected to the pressure of the body's weight and grow inward. They can become painful when they press on sensitive tissues under them. The viruses can be killed with special medications, applied to the wart, or the infected tissue can be cut out by a podiatrist. Then healthy skin grows in to fill the space that is left.

Diabetics have special foot problems. Their skin is easily infected, and it heals very slowly. So they must be especially careful to keep the feet clean and dry, to wear well-fitted shoes, and to cut the toenails properly so that ingrown toenails will not form.

74

A practice called *foot reflexology* has become popular in recent years. It is based on the idea that pains in other parts of the body are linked with defects in the feet. Reflexologists claim that crystallike deposits in the feet cause poor function and distress in various organs. By massaging the particular area of the foot linked with the organ that is giving trouble, they say, the harmful crystals can be broken up and energy can flow again to the organ, reestablishing its normal function. These claims have not been supported by objective tests, and most doctors do not believe there is anything to the theory behind them. But it is true that a good foot massage can relax you and make you feel better.

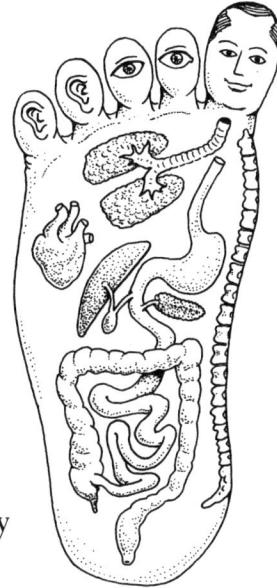

As for care of the feet themselves, the best advice seems obvious: Treat them well by keeping them clean and dry and providing them with shoes that give support without squeezing, and your feet will reward you with a lifetime of good service.

More information about foot problems and how to treat them can be found in the following books.

Block, Barry H. *Foot Talk.* New York: Zebra Books, 1985.

Sandler, Marvin. *Your Guide to Foot Care: What to Do About Your Aching Feet.* Philadelphia: Stickley, 1984.

Schneider, Myles and Mark Sussman. *How to Doctor Your Feet Without a Doctor.* Washington, D.C.: Acropolis Books, 1984.

Index

(Numbers in *italics* refer to illustrations.)

abductor digiti minimi, *37*
abductor hallucis, *37*
Achilles tendon, 36, 50
adductor hallucis, *37*
aerobic dancing, 62, 67
aerobic exercises, 57, 58, 59
afferent neuron, *41*
ankle, 14, *14*, 54
ankle bone, 29, 32
ankle joint, 29
ants, 8
apes, 11, 53
arch, *14*, 26, 32, 49
arch support, 68
arterial blood, 44
arteries, 43, *44*
artificial limbs, 42
athlete's foot, 73–74

Babinski's reflex, 19, *19*
balance, 51
balance organs, 49
ball of foot, 14, *14*, 18, 33, 49, 54
ballerina, 55
basketball, 59, 67
bears, 8, *9*, 53, *54*
bees, 9–10, *10*
bicycling, 59
big toe, 15, 32, 36, 38, 55

biomechanics, 61
bipeds, 8, 51, *51*
birds, 8
blister, 40, 72, *72*
blood, 43
blood clots, 23
bones of foot, 28–33, *30*, *31*
bowlegs, 64, *64*
brain, 41, 48, 53
broad jump, 55
broken bones, 69
bunions, 65, 71–72, *71*
buoyancy, 56
bursa, 71, *74*
butterflies, 9

calcaneus, 29, *30*, 33, 34
calf muscle, 34, 36
calluses, 18, 70
capillaries, 43, 44, 45, 47
carbon dioxide, 44
carpals, 32
cartilage, 31, *31*
cats, 10, 54
center of gravity, 49, 50
cerebellum, 41
cerebrum, 41
chimpanzees, 8
circulation, 45

clams, 9
claws, 10
club foot, 26, *26*
collagen, 17
"cooling down" period, 58
coordination of movement, 41
corneal layer, 16
corns, 70–71, *71*
cuboid, 29, *30*, 33
cuneiforms, 29, *30*
cuts, 69

dermis, 17, 20, 22
development of foot, 68
diabetes, 24, 74
digitigrade, 54, *54*
dog, 54, *54*
dominant foot, 15

ears, 49
efferent neuron, *41*
elastic fibers, 17
elephants, 54, *55*
epidermis, 16, 17, 20, 23
evolution of foot, 8
exercise, 56–59
extensor digitorum longus, *35*
extensor hallucis longus, *35*
extensor muscles, 34

fainting, 46
fat pads, 17, 26
feedback, 39, 53
feet, functions of, 7–8, 9–10
feet, size of, 13, 15
feet, structure of, 13–15
fibula, 29
fire walking, 42–43
fitness, 56

fitting shoes, 66, *66*
flat foot, *20*, 64, *65*, 68
flea, 55–56, *56*
flexor digiti minimi brevis, *37*
flexor digitorum brevis, *37*
flexor digitorum longus, *37*
flexor hallucis brevis, *37*
flexor hallucis longus, *37*
flexor muscles, 34
fly, 10
foot, development of, 68
foot, structure of, 28–36, *30*, *31*,
    33, *35*, *37*
foot binding, 26–27, *27*
foot bones, 28
foot-hands, 11, 13
foot problems, 69–75
foot reflexology, 75
football, 60
footprints, 20, *20*
fossils, 12, 54
fracture, 69
Franklin, Tony, 61
frog, 56
frostbite, 47
fungus infection, 24, 73

gastrocnemius muscle, 34, *35*,
    36, 38, 50
giraffe, 55, *55*
gliding joints, 29, 31, *31*
gorillas, 8, *9*
gravity, 48, 56

hair, 16, 22
hair follicle, *16*, 17, 22
hammertoe, 71, *71*
hand, similarities of foot to, *30*,
    31–32

heart, 44
heel, 14, *14*, 17, 18, 24, 49, 53,
    54, *55*, *74*
heel bone, 29, 33, 34, 36
heel pad, 68
heel spurs, 73, *74*
high heels, 50, *50*, 65
hinge joints, 14, 29, 31, *31*
hippos, 54
hoofed mammals, 54
horse, 55, *55*
houseflies, 8, 9
human, *54*

identical twins, 20
infant, 24
ingrown toenails, 73, *73*, 74
injuries, 62–63
insects, 8, 50
instep, 14, *14*, 36, 61

jogging, 58, 62, 67
joint capsule, 31, *31*
jumping, 38, 55, 56, *56*

kangaroos, 8, *9*, 10, 56
keratin, 16, 22, 23
kicking, 10, 15, 56, 60–61, *60*
knock-knee, 64, *64*, 68
knuckle walking, 9

lateral arch, 32, *33*
leaping, 55
leather shoes, 21
legs, number of, 8
lever action, 28, 38, *38*
ligaments, 28, *31*, 69, 70
lion, *54*
little toe, 15, 36, 38

locomotion, *51*
"lotus foot", 26
lung cancer, 24
lymph capillaries, 44
lymphatics, *44*, 45

mammals, 8
massage, 75
matrix, 24
medial arch, 32, *33*
melanin, 22
metatarsals, 29, *30*, 33
millipedes, 8
monkeys, 11, *11*, 53
motor nerves, 40
muscle strains, 61
muscles, 28, 34, *35*, *37*, 40, 48,
    70
muscles of foot, 34–38, *35*, *37*,
    38

nail bed, 23, *23*
nail plate, *23*
nail root, 22
nails, 16
navicular, 29, *30*
nerve, *16*, 39
neutral position, 49, 68

orthopedic shoes, 67
orthotics, 68
oxygen, 57

pain, 7, 40, 63, 64
pain receptors, 39, 43
papillae, 17, 20
papillary ridges, 20
paralysis, 42
parrots, 10

Pepke, Allen, 62
peroneus brevis, *35*
peroneus longus, *37*
peroneus tertius, *35*
phalanges, 29, 33
phalanx, 29, *30*
phantom sensations, 42
pigs, 54
pins and needles, 19
pirouette, 55
plantar fascia, 73, *74*
plantar reflex, 19, *19*
plantar wart, 74, *74*
plantigrade, 53, *54*
podiatrist, 63
pointed-toe shoes, 65–66
polio, 42
pooling of blood, 46
posture, 50, *50*
prehumans, 12
pressure problems, 70
pronation, 64, *64*, 65
psoriasis, 24
pulse rate, 57, *57*, 58
pumping action of leg muscles, 45
puncture wound, 69

quadrupeds, 51, *51*

raccoons, 10
racewalking, 52, 58
radiation, 47
rash, 63
Raynaud's syndrome, 47
reflex, 19
reflex actions, 40
reflex arc, *41*
reptiles, 8

rhinoceros, 54
R.I.C.E. (Rest, Ice, Compression, Elevation), 69–70
ridges, 24
runners, 23
running, 51, *51*, 52, 54
running shoes, 67

saddle joint, 32
scissors grip, 32
sebaceous gland, *16*, 17, 22
Seltzer, Richard, 23
sense organs, 9
sense receptors, *16*, 17, 18, 53
sensory nerves, 39
Shepherd, Cybill, 27
shock absorption, 18, 33, 53
shoes, 27, 38, 55, 58, 61, 64, 65–67, *66*, *67*, 70, 71, 72
skeleton, 48, *49*
skin, 15–21
smelly feet, 21
snail, 9, *9*
sneakers, 73
soccer, 60
sole, 14, *14*, 17, 18, 19, 20, 22, 26, 39, 43, 64, 73
soleus, 36
spiders, 8, *9*
spinal cord, 40, 42
spinal column, 48, *49*
sprain, 69, 70
squirrels, 10
stamina, 59
step, 32–33, 52–53, *52*, *53*, 65
Stepanov, Yuri, 38
strain, 70
stretching exercises, 58
subcutaneous tissue, 17

suntan, 22
supination, 64, *64*, 65
"sway back", 50
sweat glands, *16*, 17, 20
sweat pores, 21
sweating, 21
swimming, 56, 59
swollen feet, 46

talus, 29, *30*, 32
tarsals, 32, 33
temperature regulation, 46–47
temperature sense, 39
tendons, 34, 36, 70
tennis, 59, 67
tetanus, 69
thumb, 32
tibia, 29
tibialis anterior, *35*, 42
tibialis posterior, *37*
tickle, 40
toe bones, 29

toenails, 15, 23, *23*, 24
toenails, care of, 24
toes, 13–14, *14*, 15, 19, 32, 36,
    38, 54, 60
touch, 39
transverse arch, 32, *33*
traumatic injuries, 69
tuberculosis, 24
"tuned" track, 61

ungulates, 55, *55*

valves, 45, *45*
veins, 44, *44*
viruses, 74

walking, 24, 50–55, *51*, *52*, *53*,
    57
willow walk, 26, 27
wrist bones, 32

X ray, 31